Ah-Choo!

Ah-Choo!

The Uncommon Life of
Your Common Cold

JENNIFER ACKERMAN

TWELVE

New York   Boston

Twelve
Hachette Book Group
237 Park Avenue
New York, NY 10017

www.HachetteBookGroup.com

Twelve is an imprint of Grand Central Publishing.
The Twelve name and logo are trademarks of Hachette Book
Group, Inc.

Printed in the United States of America

First Edition: September 2010
10 9 8 7 6 5 4 3 2 1

Library of Congress Cataloging-in-Publication Data
Ackerman, Jennifer.
Ah-choo! : The uncommon life of your common cold / Jennifer
Ackerman.—1st ed.
p. cm.
Includes index.
ISBN 978-0-446-54115-2
1. Cold (Disease)—Popular works.   I. Title.
RF361.A25 2010
616.2'05—dc22
2010004794

*To Melanie Jackson
with warm thanks for twenty years
of friendship and wise counsel*

"A family unit is composed not only of children but of men, women, an occasional animal, and the common cold."

OGDEN NASH

CONTENTS

Ah-Choo!

THE COLD TRUTH

It's like so many pivotal points in life: the moment milk turns from sweet to sour, or a toddler's cheery mood tips into tantrum. One minute you're yourself, perhaps with a faint scratch in the back of the throat, nothing alarming. The next you're a vessel of full-blown congestive fury and malaise. Do you know what it is to succumb to such "an insurmountable day-mare? An indisposition to do anything or to be anything; a total deadness and distaste; a suspension of vitality; an indifference to locality; a numb, soporifical good-for-nothingness; an ossification all over; an oyster-like insensibility to the passing events; a mind-stupor? Did you ever have a very bad cold?"

To Charles Lamb's bleating question, the vast majority of us can answer a resounding yes.

Wally Schirra certainly could. As commander of Apollo 7, the first manned mission after the fiery Apollo 1 launchpad disaster, Schirra shot into space in 1968 only to develop one of the most debilitating and famous colds in American history. About an hour after liftoff and only six hours after his prelaunch physical examination, Schirra experienced one of those transitional moments when a cold suddenly launched. The minor throat irritation rapidly evolved into clogging congestion and what on Earth would have been a raging runny nose. In weightless space, however, the mucus just hung about, filling his nose and sinuses; the only relief was forceful nose blowing, which battered his eardrums. Soon Schirra's fellow crewmen, too, had succumbed to the virulent bug, and the three men hurtled through space grumpy, distracted, barely able to breathe or hear. Schirra's daughter called the flight the "ten-day cold capsule." The crewmen all returned to Earth safely, but none ever soared into space again. Their commander later appeared on TV ads for the decongestants used during the flight, holding up a space helmet and asking, "You ever sneeze in one of these?"

That decisive turning point, that moment a cold virus gains entrance and takes hold in the body, occurs in each of us as many as 200 times over a lifetime. Maybe you're down with one now, cursing that croupy little cough, filling your trash bin with soggy tissues. This book tells the story of a malady so universal its very name reflects its frequency. (Though when it strikes the high and mighty, it may bear the self-important moniker "executive flu.") Why should we care about this petty plague? A single cold is, of course, mostly a minor annoyance. But if you take a moment to calculate just how much suffering this run-of-the-mill bug inflicts over a normal life span, you'll see that it amounts to some five years of congestion, coughing, headache, sore throat—and roughly a full year in bed. Wouldn't it be a good idea to get a grip on such a relentlessly regular visitor, to take a healthy interest in this unhealthy interloper?

Viewed from a distance, there's a lot about the common cold that defies common sense. Its name, for instance. The cold may be common but it's still a little black hole of an ailment, ill understood. Moreover, talk as we might of "the" common cold, no single agent causes it but rather an army of different agents. And why "cold"? Because we feel chilly when we have one? Or because it occurs more often in the colder seasons? While it's true that colds most often strike in cooler, wetter weather, any link to low temperatures is tenuous at best. Yet in many languages, the word for the ailment faithfully mirrors the word for coolness—*raffreddore* in Italian (from the Latin *frigidus*); *resfriado* in Portuguese; *erkältung* in German—to catch a cold or a chill.

Why is the common cold still so common? The long, fruitless search for a cure made one cold research center the butt of British humor. A cartoon shows an elderly scientist in the laboratory at the Common Cold Unit in Salisbury, England, putting his arm around a younger scientist, saying, "I know, I know! There's no glamour in this branch of science, young man—but at least it's a permanent job!" If we can vanquish killer viruses such as polio, why in the world is there no vaccine or cure for the common cold?

Why are some colds like mice, timid and irritating; others like Lamb's dragon, dragging us deep into miserable malaise for days at a time? Why do some people seem maddeningly resistant to colds while others seem to succumb after just seeing someone sneeze?

What is a cold, anyway? Can you actually "fight one off"? Which remedies really work, and which are hoaxes?

Scientists call this the golden age of the cold for good reason. For one thing, the odious cold is as prevalent as ever—perhaps more so. Children in this country get as many as 12 colds a year; adults, 2 to 4. (How many you get as an adult often hinges on whether you're exposed to children, who are often described as the "major reservoirs of cold virus.") Modern society, it seems, has created an ideal environment for colds to jump from nose to nose. Globalization and the transfer of most work to the indoors means that we share more spaces and surfaces with other people than ever before. Our offices, gyms, and public spaces, where large numbers of people work and play shoulder to shoulder, are viral swapping grounds. Our day-care centers and elementary schools, where children cluster to share secretions, are cold-breeding swamps. "Not since the trenches of World War I have germs been as efficiently shared as in today's child care centers," writes Harley Rotbart, M.D., vice chairman of pediatrics at the University of Colorado Denver School of Medicine.

This is also a golden age of understanding. What we've learned over the past decade or so has revolutionized our view of colds—what they are, what they do to our bodies, how to stifle them, and whether it's wise to do so. The common cold as a medical quest may seem low on the list of priorities compared with the more dire threats of cancer, heart disease, diabetes, and obesity. After all, a cold has never killed anyone. (Or has it?) Why would medical research dally with such an apparently dilettantish disease? When I started work on this book, my editor asked, "Would I have to travel all the way to Wales to meet a credible cold expert?" He had once commissioned a book on the quest to cure baldness, which turned out to be a very short book indeed, he said, because the author discovered that no medical researcher worth his salt would devote his time to the hair-loss issue when so many serious diseases needed to be treated.

Not so with the cold. There's a whole department full of credible cold researchers right down the road from me at the University of Virginia Medical Center, busily harvesting fresh cold virus from the noses of cold-ridden donors and smearing the virus-laden secretions on telephones and light switches, computer keyboards, and refrigerators. They're delivering cold viruses directly to the nares of willing volunteers. They're observing the nose-picking habits of doctors and medical students. They're scooping up stuffed animals from the toy bins of pediatricians' offices and TV remotes from homes and hotel rooms to sleuth for the presence of cold virus and testing nasal sprays, lotions, and cleaning products designed to abolish it.

The reason they're so engaged?

Americans catch as many as a billion colds a year and spend billions of dollars on medications to treat them. (Peering into the medicine cabinet of the average American household, which lodges up to eight different cold remedies, reveals that stuffy noses and coughs are a big deal indeed.) Getting a cold may be common, but it isn't cheap. Each year in this country, colds account for up to 100 million doctor visits, more than 1.5 million trips to the emergency room, and hundreds of millions of absences from work, with an estimated economic burden of $60 billion in the United States alone. Colds cause more illness in children than all other diseases combined and are responsible for 189 million missed days of school, up to half of school absences. Then there's the matter of colds that exacerbate other diseases and even kill—and some of them, it turns out, most certainly do. Finally, what we may learn from cold viruses—how to prevent them and halt their spread—may have implications for controlling pandemic flu.

In exploring the cold's fertile turf, science has unearthed some surprises. No two colds are alike, for instance. And you don't have to be "run down" to catch one. As Jack Gwaltney Jr., professor emeritus at the University of Virginia School of Medicine and arguably one of the world's foremost experts on the cold, has said, "The greatest myth about the common cold is that susceptibility requires a weakened immune system." If you're keen on tamping down a cold, "boosting" your immunity may be the last thing you want to do. And perhaps most unexpected: If you feel like cursing the day-care center that's efficiently delivering one cold virus after another to your darling daughter, hold your horses. There could be a silver lining to her red nose. If we were ever to banish cold bugs altogether, we might find that we actually miss them—in more ways than one.

Chapter 1

IN COLD PURSUIT

One Monday in October, against the counsel of friends, I applied to catch a cold. Five weeks later, on Friday, the 13th of November, tucked away on the seventh floor of a three-star hotel, I open up my nose to assault by a virus and wait.

It's the peak of the swine flu epidemic. Colleagues, friends, and family are succumbing one after another to the feverish misery of H1N1. After weeks of scrupulously avoiding the sniffling masses, I actually invite infection, opting to join a select group of subjects taking part in a cold study at the University of Virginia. The plan is to check in to a local hotel on a Friday afternoon, have a common strain of cold virus injected into the nose, and then hunker down for the weekend, waiting for cold symptoms to develop.

My family thinks I've gone off the deep end. My plan elicits this merry note from my dour sister: "You know our family. It'll go straight to your chest." One friend dubs it my weekend "frolic at the rhinovirus festival." "Chin up!" he says. "That way your nose won't drip." Another friend takes a darker view.

"I'll keep you in my prayers: Death by cold is one of my greatest anxieties."

Death by cold?

It's a strange thing to anticipate even mild illness, to know that in a few days viral lightning will strike. It's like awaiting the arrival of a massive snowstorm or a hurricane. There's that sense of urgency, of the need to get things done before you're under the weather and not feeling like doing much more than hanging around in your bathrobe, nursing a cup of hot tea. What kind of people normally go in for this form of weekend entertainment? As far as I can tell, mostly young male students.

The researchers have set up shop in Room 726. Oddly enough, there are no signs in the lobby, "WELCOME VIRUS STUDY SUBJECTS!" But when I reach the seventh floor, the hall is lined with boys and their backpacks in cold pursuit of three free meals a day, a clean bed, and a $600 fee. I look around for one young man I met earlier at the screening for this study, a big guy with tattoos and what sounded like serious congestion. The screening took place at around 9 a.m. on a Monday morning. When the nurse asked this fellow if he had a cold, he said no, he wasn't sick; he had just been "playing outside in the cold all morning, since 3:30 a.m."

Oh, and what was the game?

"Setting traps for animals."

There are a few outliers. As we're checking in with the study nurse, I ask the middle-aged woman in line ahead of me whether her family thinks she's crazy to be participating in this study. "Oh no," she says cheerily. "In fact, I've brought my 18-year-old daughter"—the dark-haired beauty sitting with the nurse to the right of us, awaiting the results of the routine pregnancy test. "This will take care of Christmas. My husband would have come, too, but he works for Student Health, and that created some kind of conflict of interest." A couple of years ago, she joined another such study in order to give her daughter a bang-up sweet sixteen party.

With the help of willing subjects such as these, researchers can probe the basics of a disease and also try out remedies. At a hotel up the road from ours, similar studies produced the flu drugs Relenza and Tamiflu. The flu studies are the really lucrative gigs. Nine days of isolation in a hotel room with a nasty case of flu will net you $1,750. One such opportunity recently drew a married couple who participated sequentially. First the wife got the flu (while the husband cared for their three boys) and then her spouse did. This—18 days of combined illness—so the whole family could take a $3,500 vacation.

It's money hard earned. There's the sledgehammer of the flu itself. Then there's the isolation in a hotel room. Nine days is a long time in one room, even under perfect conditions. And conditions are not always perfect. Once, lightning struck the hotel, and the electricity went out for three days. No lights, no television, no coffee pot. The hotel staff had to carry food for 80 subjects up five flights of stairs from the kitchen in the basement; meals were a little less than punctual and a lot less than hot. For entertainment, younger subjects resorted to saving up their fruit from dinner and bowling with it in the halls.

Another time, a fire in the elevator shaft prompted a hotel-wide evacuation. The study participants stood around in the icy parking lot in their slippers and pajamas, wearing masks, while the rest of the hotel guests gawked.

Our three-day stay is easy by comparison. Still, it feels strangely surreal, like a hybrid of holiday, hospital, and prison. During these three days, we can't leave the hotel for any reason (unless we drop out of the study and forsake our fee), which prompts young Tom Jackson in the room next door to mutter from his doorway, "I feel like I'm in *The Shining*." We're not even supposed to wander down to the end of the floor, where regular guests are lodged (one would hope at a deep discount). And, of course, we have to submit to a litany of nasal exams, nasal washes, and nasal sprays at all hours of the day and night.

This study is testing the effects of a new nasal spray, one of the latest shining hopes of cold treatment. The spray contains a synthetic version of a compound the body's own immune system uses to kill microbes. In this nasal form, it's designed to murder a virus before it can do its dirty work in the nose. But it's also effective against bacteria and fungi and has been used effectively as a treatment for conjunctivitis and impetigo. The study is carefully designed as a so-called randomized, placebo-controlled, double-blind experiment. Half of us picked at random will get spritzed with the real McCoy, the active-ingredient spray; half with a placebo saline spray. No one knows which group they're in; not even the scientists conducting the study—hence the expression "double blind." I'm secretly hoping the roll of the dice put me in the placebo group; I'm not sure I want up my nose what may turn out to double as a cure for toe fungus.

After we're settled into our rooms, the study's chief investigator, Birgit Winther, in white lab coat and blue gloves, comes around to infect us. Winther is an associate professor of otolaryngology (often called ENT for ear, nose, and throat) at the University of Virginia and a pioneer in cold research. Not long ago, she and her colleague Owen Hendley revealed the deeply disappointing news that guests checking out of hotel rooms leave behind more than just loose change. Their now-infamous hotel studies showed that people with colds may bestow little deposits of cold viruses on surfaces throughout a room and that these germs linger long after the sniffling guest is gone.

Winther asks me to lie with my head hanging over the foot of my hotel bed and administers the virus in a saline suspension, two sprays per nostril. It's not unlike a nasal vaccine, she tells me. It's produced the same way, with all of the safety precautions, except that it contains a live virus, a common strain of cold virus in experimental form. Into the nose is the ideal way to deliver the bug for the same reason it's a good avenue for vaccines: it offers the most direct route to the body's immune response. "The nose is set up to sample viruses that come in from the outside and to alert the immune system," Winther explains.

The common cold is caused by at least 200 different viruses. The experimental one now making its way through my nasal passages—affectionately known as T39—belongs to the largest family, the rhinoviruses, which account for 40 percent of all colds. There are at least five families of cold viruses, among them the picornaviruses (which includes rhinoviruses), adenoviruses, coronaviruses, parainfluenza viruses, and influenza viruses. Yes, *those* influenza viruses. Something like 15 percent of colds are caused by flu viruses. (This gave me pause once, when I was considering deliberately catching a cold from a friend in order to participate in another cold study. What if she was infected by something more insidious than a simple rhinovirus?) With this many flavors, you can catch one new cold virus after another and never run out—which is precisely what happens. After your body encounters a particular strain of virus and mounts a proper immune response, it dutifully produces antibodies to that virus, which will disable that strain the next time you're exposed to it. But this still leaves you susceptible to the hundreds of other remaining circulating strains. That colds are caused by this enormous menagerie of cold bugs is what has made creating a vaccine thus far impossible.

As Winther injects the cold-virus solution into my nostrils, I imagine the little beasties getting straight to work. The nose has virtually no protection against the virus once it is deposited on the nasal mucosa. Nearly everyone exposed to a cold virus in this direct fashion will get infected, provided they don't have antibodies. (And none of the study subjects do. We were tested earlier for the presence of antibodies to this strain and found wanting—which means that our bodies have never been exposed to it.)

But here's the weird thing: Though all the members of our study group will get infected and none of us has immunity to this virus, only 75 percent of us will actually come down with a cold. The other 25 percent will have virus growing in our noses but will get off pretty much scot-free, with no symptoms—whether or not we receive treatment. This is what's known as asymptomatic infection. Why some people get infected and never suffer symptoms (but still make antibodies) while others experience the full knock-down, drag-out syndrome of a cold seems utterly illogical, and it's one of the great mysteries gripping cold science. "We really don't know why this is," says Winther, "but it could be the key to colds"—why we get them and how we can avoid them. "There are so many things we still don't know about the common cold," Winther remarks later. "As a mother with children, I think we deserve a better understanding."

Just a tiny smack of rhinovirus—as little as a single particle—is enough to give you an infection. But just to be sure, the saline solution Winther delivers contains 100 particles. These experimental buggers are getting a free ride. Normally, rhinoviruses have to steal into your nasal passages, often by way of a contaminated finger probing a nose or rubbing an eye. It was Winther and her team who discovered that cold viruses can travel down the lacrimal (or tear) duct from the eye into the nose. There, they encounter the thick, sticky mucus lining your nasal passages, which traps viruses and other foreign particles before they enter the lungs. Some viruses inevitably escape this viscous barrier and travel on to the big lymph glands known as adenoids at the back of your throat.

Oddly enough, they're assisted in their journey by the nose itself. Cells lining the nasal passage carry tiny hairs that beat vigorously in unison, driving the mucus that coats them. Under a scanning electron microscope, these hairs look like nothing so much as a shag carpet. Normally, they act as a kind of nasal hausfrau, sweeping dust, pollen, and other particles toward the back of the throat to be swallowed and destroyed by the acids of the stomach. But the tiny hairs can also act like a little moving sidewalk for the virus, bearing it toward the back of the nose.

Within some 10 to 15 minutes, the rhinoviruses are deposited in the nasopharynx, what the 19th-century physician Sir William Osler called the "garbage dump" of the throat. There, in the soft tissue of the adenoids (aptly described as "crypts"), the tiny invaders approach body cells a thousand times their size, like pirates in a small speedboat approaching an oil tanker. They get onboard by wily means, pretending to be something they're not. (Coast Guard? Tourists?) Cold viruses have evolved a specialized device for docking on a target host cell: little canyonlike grooves on their surface that fit perfectly with specialized receptors on the surface of your body cells (called ICAM-1 receptors). The fit is tight, like lock and key.

Once the virus particles are docked, the sedition begins. They fool a body cell into thinking they're something useful, so the cell readily takes them in. And once they're onboard, like pirates, they take over the controls. That is, unless you're lucky enough to have been exposed to this strain of virus before and possess antibodies against it. In that case, the antibodies neutralize the viral particles by binding to their surface, obstructing their ability to dock with your body cells. Otherwise, the virus slips into the jelly of a cell and releases its little stitch of genetic material, RNA. The RNA hijacks the machinery of your own cells, using it to produce hundreds of copies of the virus. Eventually your body cell starts to destroy itself, and the mother lode of fresh virus particles is released to infect surrounding cells.

This part of the infection is the genesis of that scratchy sore throat that so often heralds a cold, the uncomfortable feeling like a pair of pants too tight at the waist or the faintly itchy sensation of a wool sweater on a warm day.

"From the time a cold virus enters your nose, it takes around 8 to 12 hours for the virus to complete its reproductive cycle and for new cold virus to be released into nasal secretions," says Ron Turner, a cold expert and colleague of Winther's at the University of Virginia. This is what's known as the incubation period.

You have to admire how something so small and so simple can be so ingenious. "Rhinovirus infection is not only very efficient, it proceeds very rapidly," says Turner. Only 24 hours after a single virus particle enters your nose, *Bam!* Infected cells have been coerced into making millions of new viruses, which are then sent out to infect other healthy cells. The sneezing, snuffling misery tends to begin within 12 hours of infection but typically peaks at around 48 to 72 hours.

At the hotel, nurses knock on our doors three times a day to monitor our symptoms: any fever, sneezing, runny nose, nasal obstruction, sore or scratchy throat, cough, headache, feverishness, chilliness, malaise. We sit in chairs in our hotel room doorways like unadopted pets at the pound. From the chatter, it's clear there's some confusion about the nature of the bugs now flourishing in our noses. They're not bacteria, as some of the boys seem to think, but viruses. This is why antibiotics have no effect on colds. Zip. Nil. Antibiotics kill bacteria by preventing them from building their cell walls. Viruses are not cells and have no cell walls, so they're utterly unaffected by the drugs. This is also why those antibacterial soaps, shampoos, and lotions have no effect on cold germs. Promotional claims notwithstanding, these products will do nothing to protect you, your friends, or your family from contracting a cold.

After the first 12 hours, most of us are still symptom-free. (Come to think of it, I do feel a kind of creeping crumminess. But that might be on account of having our nasal spray delivered late last night and then again at 6:30 this morning.)

Early on the morning of the second day, I take an informal survey of my fellow patients and hear about a range of complaints, from mild to severe. Colds don't usually cause fever in adults, but some subjects tell me they are registering a "normal" 98.6 degrees Fahrenheit in the morning. This is in fact not a normal morning temperature. Body temperature varies over the course of the day by as much as two degrees Fahrenheit. It's lowest in the morning, usually around 97 degrees or so, and rises to as high as 99 degrees in the evening. So at 6:30 a.m., a temperature registering 98.6 degrees could actually be considered a low-grade fever.

What do the study participants view as the worst of cold symptoms? Some can't abide that heraldic sore throat at the start of a cold that sabotages swallowing—with its sharp reminder every time our throat opens and closes. Others despise the congestion and runny nose that blocks or floods the harbor of our nostrils, disrupting the sweet pleasures of breathing and tasting. Many are dreading the impending cough that annihilates sleep.

This is what makes colds so irritating and distracting—they

make those basic body functions of which we're normally blissfully unaware suddenly leap into unpleasant consciousness.

The sore, scratchy throat that makes a trial of downing spit results when the body sends blood rushing to the infected cells at the back of the throat, releasing chemicals that make the blood vessels in the surrounding tissue swell. The swelling pressures nerve endings in the throat, causing pain every time you do what you have to do so you won't choke on your own saliva. (Lest you think we're the only species that suffers so, a new study suggests that the seven-ton *Tyrannosaurus rex* at the Field Museum in Chicago, nicknamed Sue, actually died of a sore throat. Scientists suspect that a parasite that also infects pigeons made it difficult for the dinosaur to swallow, leading to starvation. So we're in splendid company.)

Rarely do colds produce lasting throat soreness. But neither is it a temporary, acute pain, like a hammer blow to the thumb. This is unfortunate, as it means that for sore throats, we can't call on what science tells us is an accessible and convenient form of painkiller for acute pain, such as stove burn or stubbed toe: swearing. A 2009 study at Keele University's School of Psychology in England found that channeling your inner sailor can actually diminish pain. Swearing, it seems, triggers both an emotional and a physical response that together raise heart rate and reduce pain. Alas, it's more effective for the sudden, hammer-nailing-thumb sort of hurt than the swollen grip of a sore throat. The only real relief for the latter comes from the messier but less profane remedy of a saltwater gargle. (But more on that later.)

As for congestion: The job of the nose is nothing less than making air fit for your lungs to breathe. It's hardly a simple task. Air flows into the nose not in a straightforward rivulet but in whirls and eddies more complex than the airstream over the wings of a plane or blood flow through the heart, while the nose warms, filters, and humidifies it. No wonder we suffer when a cold runs interference. Our mouths are not nearly as deft at air-conditioning. And since 75 percent of flavor is aroma, a blocked sense of smell obliterates taste—among the most egregious of a cold's sins, at least in my book. (Also in Charles Lamb's. "I inhale suffocation," wrote poor, cold-ridden Lamb. "I can't distinguish veal from mutton.")

But don't blame mucus for the nasal blockage. The problem is more fundamental.

Or architectural.

There's a sort of Roman nobility to the nose, both inside and out. Its interior is composed of two large air passages, separated by the thin wall of the septum. These passages lead to four sinus cavities just above, behind, and below your eyes. Spongy shelves called turbinates line the sidewalls of the nasal passages and help trap particles entering the nose. They also heat and humidify the air so it's warm and almost completely saturated with moisture by the time it reaches the lungs.

The stuffy, blocked feeling that stifles breathing during a cold is not the product, as one might expect, of excess mucus but the result of swelling blood vessels in the turbinates. The turbinates are designed to engorge this way, just like other erectile tissues in the body. They normally swell in a rhythmic, alternating cycle—first one side, then the other—so that one nasal passage always has a little less airflow than the other. It's not clear why they do this, but the cycling may rest one nasal chamber while the other fulfills the duty of air-conditioning. Colds tend to exaggerate the asymmetry of the rhythm, completely closing one nasal passage, so breathing becomes a labored affair. Though the urge is great to forcefully expel whatever's causing the blockage with a good hard snort, one should try to resist the temptation. Blowing out the mucus isn't going to make your nose feel less stuffy. And you don't particularly want to blow out your turbinates, even if you could.

Though it has not yet shown up as a symptom among my cold compatriots, within a few days, coughing may be the bane of many on this sick hall. First, there's the quick inspiration of breath, followed by an involuntary squeeze of the diaphragm. The glottis—that cap on the larynx at the back of the throat—suddenly pops open, releasing a turbulent blast of air from the lungs traveling at more than 80 feet per second. Coughing is a reflex that protects the airways in the throat and chest. It helps to eject any foreign substance that might be tickling the larynx or the trachea (the tube leading to your lungs). Its sound depends on the site of irritation. The barking seal sound of croup, for instance, arises from an irritated voice box.

Naturally, it's a good idea to eject foreign matter. But when you have a cold, the chemicals your body produces may continuously tickle the nerve endings in the larynx or trachea, making them think there's something there—phantom foreign material—to expel. Coughing becomes, as Ogden Nash once wrote, "like the steps of a moving stair, there is always another cough there."

By day three, I have most of the usual early symptoms, as do about half of the study participants. And my dour sister was right—the blasted bug will eventually give me a chest cough that's hard to shake. This scientifically induced cold may have been designed to be mild, but for me, it turns out to be a humdinger, and it's almost 10 days before I finally get over the residual, nagging hack.

Either there isn't much to this new nasal spray product or I and my fellow cold sufferers were the recipients of the placebo saline solution. I'm guessing it's the latter. Birgit Winther has seen a lot of drugs come and go, and she's genuinely optimistic about this new one. She likes it because it's designed to work the way the body's own compounds work to fight viruses—and does so early in the process of infection. Winther thinks it could be used prophylactically, to stave off the spread of colds in a family if a child comes home with a doozy. But it will be some time before we know whether the spray is really effective. Even if this study shows positive results, these must be confirmed by other, larger studies. As scientists are quick to point out, a single study does not a finding make. It's just a start.

Early Monday morning, everyone is packed up and sitting in the doorways to our hotel rooms, awaiting discharge. We're all keenly aware that we're about to go home with a little more microbial baggage than we had when we arrived. Colds are most contagious during the first two to four days after symptoms appear, so at this point, we're all walking Typhoid Marys. After we leave, the study staff will have to scrub our hotel rooms with alcohol and bleach to kill any critters we've left behind on sink handles, TV remotes, light switches, and phones.

They don't scrub us, but they do ask us to wash our hands.

When I hear that we're all invited for a buffet breakfast in the lobby before we leave, I make a mental note to avoid brunch at this hotel. It turns out, however, that the staff has exercised caution here, too, assigning us to a private breakfast room of our own. Still I have to wonder: How thoroughly did the boys wash up—or any of us for that matter? What are the chances of passing some residual little T39s to the waitress, along with our basket of sweet rolls or jam knife?

Just how does one normally catch cold?

Chapter 2

IT'S CATCHING

The empty conveyor belt and the curious absence of a line at the otherwise packed grocery store should have been a dead giveaway. But not until all of my groceries were unloaded did I notice the check-out clerk with the chafed and reddened nostrils. It was a few days before Christmas, and I was in a hurry. I considered swooping my piles back into the cart and hightailing it to the next line over. But it was too late; she was ringing up my milk and cheese. She looked miserable and sniffed noisily every 10 seconds or so as she plowed slowly through my pile of organic onions, potatoes, and peppers. Still, her affliction seemed harmless enough until with just a few items left in my order, she suddenly wrinkled her nose, caught her breath, turned slightly, and sneezed ferociously, sending a spray of fine droplets partly into her sleeve but mostly onto my heaping grocery bag. Then she paused to tear off a piece of paper towel and blew her nose into it with such audible force that I feared for the integrity of her sinuses. To her credit, she did take a second to spritz with hand sanitizer before reaching for my head of broccoli. However, a minute later she wiped her nose with the back of her hand, then picked up my eco-friendly bag and handed it over the counter to me, tucking into it, I feared, a bonus load of rhinoviruses.

Should I have worried? What were my risks of taking home a rapacious cold along with my broccoli rabe? Was the greatest threat that spray of sneeze or the hand swipe across the nose and onto the handle of my sack?

How do you catch a cold out in the real world?

From the look of it, not all that easily. Strange but true: colds appear to spread only grudgingly—at least compared with diseases such as tuberculosis or flu. In the early days of cold research, Sir Christopher Andrewes, the director of the Common Cold Unit (CCU) in England, found that colds rarely passed between two people, even those living in the same room. Indeed, if one roommate had a cold, the other had on average only a one-in-five chance of catching it. Andrewes had an ardent interest in how colds spread, but the apparent reluctance of the cold virus to hop from one subject's nose to another frustrated his efforts to fathom its routes. Andrewes hypothesized that perhaps the volunteers in his trials were already resistant to the viruses under study. Why not try spreading a cold in a group of people who had been isolated from their fellow men? "Hermit" types, such as long-traveling Arctic explorers, were known to be highly susceptible upon their return, apt to come down with a cold almost as soon as they rejoined civilization. So in 1950, Andrewes organized his own desert island at Eilean nan Ron, or Island of Seals, a tiny island surrounded by steep cliffs off the north coast of Scotland. He sent a group of 12 volunteers to spend 10 weeks there in complete isolation, then subjected the marooned islanders to 6 people freshly infected with colds. The results were most disappointing. As Andrewes described it, "To our astonishment and dismay not a single cold developed among our twelve islanders."

A decade later, Jack Gwaltney Jr. and his colleagues at the University of Virginia shed light on the question when they launched a 15-year study of colds in employees of the local State Farm Insurance company in Charlottesville, Virginia. The team traced the spread of individual virus types through 500 workers and discovered that they didn't typically spread among people working together in the same area of the office. It took close, prolonged contact for people to get sick. The employees were more likely to become infected at home, where they were living in close quarters with family members, snuggling with sick children, sharing everything from refrigerator handles to bath towels. ("This work led to the finding that children were usually the first to develop rhinovirus colds in the family as a result of exposure at school," says Gwaltney. "The sick child then transmitted the infection to other family members.")

The point was further demonstrated in the 1970s and '80s by a professor at the University of Wisconsin School of Medicine and a serious student of poker. Elliot C. Dick threw together groups of people, half healthy, half heavy with cold, in various situations: playing cards and talking loudly for a few hours, living together in dormitory rooms for 36 hours, giving one another a lingering kiss. Only 8 or 9 percent of the healthy people living together with infected people or kissing them came down with a cold. None of the card players did. Other studies by Dick showed that even married couples living in close contact transmitted colds to one another only 30 or 40 percent of the time.

Still, the bugs manage to move around with enough efficiency to put adults under at least twice a year, and children, up to a dozen times. So how do they do it?

Cold viruses have likely been infecting our primate tribe for millions of years. Over time, they've learned a thing or two about how to take advantage of our weaknesses and curious habits.

The seeds of spread, of course, are the virus particles ensnared in the nasal secretions of an ill person. When people have a cold, the mucus they shed harbors millions of these particles, especially in the first three days of illness, when they are most contagious. But what are the viruses' routes of travel from one victim to the next?

As Dick discovered, rhinoviruses rarely enter our bodies by way of mouth. In fact, when Dick studied married couples, he found that more than half of the saliva specimens taken from 17 sneezing, sniffling married folks contained no detectable rhinovirus. When people with colds had their moist lips swabbed, only 4 samples out of 30 yielded virus, and only in tiny quantities. Moreover, when volunteers infected with cold virus kissed cold-free volunteers for a full minute and a half, only one case of cross-infection occurred in 16 trials. Estimates suggest that it takes some 8,000 times as much virus to cause infection by way of saliva than by other routes. So as far as rhinoviruses are concerned, kissing or sharing drinks is no great hazard. However, it should be noted that other common cold bugs, such as adenovirus, as well as flu bugs, may be present in saliva, so you can't really kiss without caution.

For most cold viruses, nose and eye are the primary portals of entry. But the main route by which these doors are reached has been a matter of simmering debate, the subject of study from the hotels of Virginia to the dorms of Madison, Wisconsin.

One school of thought has proposed that cold viruses wing their way through the world by airborne means, launched by coughs and sneezes. They travel either on relatively large droplets that tend to settle out of the air quickly or in "droplet nuclei," tiny, aerosolized microbial particles, which may be inhaled by unknowing victims. This is the main route of spread for influenza viruses. Not many organisms can swing airborne transmission, but those that do spread easily. "Take tuberculosis," says Gwaltney. "Epidemics have resulted from a single common source—a sailor near a ventilation system on a destroyer, for instance, or a child on a school bus."

The other school of thought on cold transmission suggests that most cold bugs, especially rhinoviruses, trace a more plodding route, by way of contact with hands and surfaces.

The issue is nothing to sneeze at. Grasping the usual mode of cold transmission is critical for shaping strategies to interrupt it: Hand treatments and sanitizing surface wipes? Or air disinfectants and germicidal lights? It also has important implications for stopping the spread of pandemic flu.

An ingenious approach to the problem was devised by none other than James Lovelock. Best known as the author of the ecological hypothesis known as Gaia, Lovelock has always had a knack for inventions and discoveries that change the way we see the world. It was Lovelock who invented the device—a handheld electron capture detector—that revealed the presence of tiny amounts of pesticides and other harmful chemicals, providing data for Rachel Carson's *Silent Spring* and exposing the accumulation in our atmosphere of chlorofluorocarbons, or CFCs, those gases that deplete the ozone layer.

In the thick of World War II, amid fears that crowding in air-raid shelters might lead to epidemics, Lovelock was hired by the CCU in England to determine how respiratory infections spread. One obvious vehicle for transmission was the sneeze. (When it comes to spreading the cold, the unguarded sneeze is "a sanitary crime," wrote an early popular textbook on hygiene. "Possibly it may in time become a social and legal one, as has promiscuous spitting.") After all, sneezing and coughing can propel droplets at a velocity of up to 150 feet per second and a distance greater than 10 feet. Early flash photography had illuminated the clouds of fine particles shot out by a sneeze, and posters everywhere in the United Kingdom reproduced the photos with the ditty "Coughs and sneezes spread diseases."

But do they spread the common cold?

To test the sneeze theory, the creative teams at the CCU fashioned an experiment using the enclosed space of a pine wardrobe. They put a chair in the wardrobe and squeezed a volunteer into the tight space. Then they used a spray bottle filled with cold virus suspension to deliver an artificial sneeze in the direction of the subject's face. Over the ensuing five days, the exposed subject obliged by coming down with a cold.

Nonetheless, Lovelock doubted that colds were spread mainly by the airborne droplets of a sneeze. He suspected a more pedestrian route. To explore the notion, he rigged up an impressive device as a surrogate runny nose: an apparatus attached to the nose of a staff member that allowed fluid stored in a little reservoir fixed to his forehead to trickle out at about the same rate as nasal secretions would during a fairly severe cold. The fluid contained a fluorescent dye. The device was set going while the lab member spent a few hours with other people, playing bridge and eating a meal together. He wiped his nose as necessary with a handkerchief stored in his back pocket and otherwise behaved normally. When the lights were turned off, as Andrewes recounts it, a "U-V lamp revealed the horrible truth." Most of the fluorescence was on the handkerchief, to be sure, but the artificial nose secretion had also "gone around everywhere—all over his face and clothes, his food, the playing cards."

It was clear to Lovelock at least that cold viruses may well be moved about on hands and objects. (He likes to take credit for one key outgrowth of this work: the general conversion to paper tissues from the sodden cotton handkerchief, which he calls "a potent aid for organisms wishing to find a new host.")

That inanimate objects could serve as passive carriers of contagion was first noted well before the discovery of viruses, when outbreaks of smallpox were traced to shipments of imported cotton. These pathogenic way stations are sometimes known as fomites, from the Latin word for "touchwood" or "tinder." A fomite can be a coffee cup, a computer keyboard, a poker chip, a doorknob, an elevator button, an ATM—virtually any small, inanimate object that can carry pathogens. In the lingo of the field, broad surfaces like tabletops that can transfer pathogens are dubbed "environmental surfaces." Fomites and environmental surfaces become contaminated when they're smeared with body secretions or fluids or come into contact with soiled hands or virus-laden droplets generated via talking, sneezing, or coughing. Cold viruses can't multiply on a surface—they need the machinery of human cells to reproduce. However, they can remain viable on inanimate objects and surfaces for surprising lengths of time and are infectious if transported from surface to nose.

The first solid evidence for the part hands and fingers may play in cold transmission came about through serendipity. Jack Gwaltney Jr. was studying the appearance of the nasal lining in infected and uninfected subjects. He noticed that infection accidentally spread to uninfected subjects by way of a contaminated nasal speculum—an instrument used to widen the nose's openings to look within its passages. For Gwaltney, this transfer by speculum suggested a number of possible ways virus might be introduced directly into the nose through the types of intimate activities that normally take place among people.

Sure enough, Gwaltney and others soon discovered that people with colds typically carry the cold virus on their hands (most probably as a result of nose blowing or wiping) and can pass it to other hands, even after only brief hand-to-hand contact. Studies by Gwaltney's colleague Owen Hendley have shown that rhinovirus remains alive on the skin, capable of infecting another person, for at least two hours. It readily transfers from the hands of the sufferer to the hands of a potential new victim, even if the contact is brief, around 10 seconds. So when a sick person shakes someone's hand, and that person touches her nose or eye, the virus makes its happy leap.

In a recent survey, one in 10 Americans admitted to wiping their nose on their hand and then extending the hand for a handshake or reaching for a doorknob.

It was this sort of research that convinced at least one politician to cease the practice of handshaking. Not long ago, Mark Cooper, a selectman from Southbury, Connecticut, made a public announcement that he would no longer be grasping the hands of his constituents. If anyone extended a paw, he would politely decline and pass them a brochure on spreading germs.

If the nose is the primary culprit in the transmission of colds, then hands—fingertips seeded with virus—are apt accomplices. So the chain goes: hand to hand (or hand to surface to hand) and thence to nose.

But surely people do not touch their noses that often.

Based on Lovelock's field observations of travelers in the London Underground, they most certainly do. And it's not just the middling masses who frequently finger their nares. Mark Nicas, a professor at the University of California, Berkeley, School of Public Health, recently videotaped 10 students working alone in an office for three hours and found that they touched their hands to their eyes, nose, and lips an average of 16 times an hour; about five of these touches were aimed at the nostril. Three subjects fiddled with and picked their noses close to 30 times in the three-hour period. (I was pleased to learn that there's actually a technical name for such habitual nose picking: rhinotillexomania, from *rhinos*, nose; *tillesthai*, to pull; and *exo*, out.)

Even health-care workers are not immune to the practice. Owen Hendley and his colleagues at the University of Virginia secretly observed physicians and other medical staff during a one-hour grand-rounds lecture in a medical school amphitheater and discovered that a third rubbed their eyes and a third picked their noses at least once during the surveillance period. The team also observed people in a Sunday school class and reported that nose picking was less frequent in the Sunday school than in the amphitheater. (I am not making this up.)

It's worth lingering for a moment on the topic of nostril excavation, as it's a touchy subject for many parents who rue the behavior in their children (and maybe in themselves). Science has only recently begun to seriously probe the matter. In 2001, two researchers from the National Institute of Mental Health in Bangalore, India, sought to remedy the paucity of world literature on nose-picking behavior in the general population. They studied 200 adolescents in four urban schools and found that almost the entire sample admitted to nose picking roughly four times a day. Thirty-four students thought they had a serious nose-picking problem. The scientists' mining of the issue won them an Ig Nobel award in Medicine, that prize for "science that first makes you laugh—and then makes you think." (Fellow award winners that year included a study on "injuries due to falling coconuts," "a partial solution to the question of why shower curtains billow inwards," and an invention for airtight underwear with a replaceable charcoal filter that removes odors from gases before they escape.) The study concluded that "nose picking may merit closer epidemiologic and nosologic scrutiny."

Indeed.

It seems most nose picking arises from the feeling that something in the nasal arena is not quite right. Children with allergies may have this feeling more than others because of the persistent cycle of mucus and crusting. Truly excessive nose picking may indicate anxiety, autism, or Asperger's disorder. But in most instances, the habit is innocuous.

In fact, Gwaltney says that it may even serve a purpose. Material deposited in the nasal vestibule, the opening of the nose, doesn't get swept into the so-called mucociliary escalator and safely delivered to the back of the throat, where it can be swallowed. "It just sits there," says Gwaltney. "So maybe nature designed the nose so that you can easily pick out this material that wouldn't otherwise be cleared."

In any case, it may calm parents to learn that young children tend to give up the habit by the time they reach school. Experts suggest offering a tissue as a substitute or swaddling the offending finger with an adhesive bandage or just keeping little hands busy with other activities. Older children may respond to gentle humor: "Give me a wave when you get to the bridge!" Above all, don't make a big deal of it, and the behavior will likely go away on its own.

The champions of viral flight as a means of cold transmission have also gone to great lengths to tout their own theory (or disprove their rival's). Airborne-transmission enthusiast Elliot Dick once devised a convincing if bizarre experiment that seemed to rule out the role of touch and fomites in transmitting colds. Dick's group asked subjects to play poker together for a full 12 hours at round tables. Two dozen of the subjects were cold donors; three dozen were susceptible healthy recipients. Half of the recipients were fitted with arm braces that allowed them to play cards but not touch their faces; others wore a plastic collar three feet in diameter (not unlike those Elizabethan collars we put on dogs to prevent them from licking their own wounds), which left their hands free but prevented them from touching eyes or nose. Despite these restraints, the bugs did their dirty work, infecting more than half to two-thirds of the susceptible folks. This suggested to Dick that the virus had to be traveling by air, as self-inoculation was impossible.

But the team did not stop there. It then convinced a dozen additional healthy volunteers to play poker with chips, cards, and pencils that were literally "gummy" with contaminated secretions from cold-stricken donors. The subjects were instructed to handle the poker paraphernalia for an hour before they were replaced with freshly contaminated ones and to make hand-to-nose contact every 15 minutes, with much rubbing of nasal and conjunctival mucosa. After 12 hours of playing, the cards were "grossly contaminated" and "soggy," but no virus could be found on the recipients' hands, and none of them came down with a cold. This suggested to the researchers that transmission of rhinoviruses by way of fomites was quite unlikely.

To quantify just how unlikely, Dick later methodically documented the near disappearance of rhinoviruses along a finger-to-fomite-to-finger-to-finger (as a stand-in for nose) contact chain. "Even though the donor may initially have thousands of infectious particles on his hands, few are deposited on fomites," wrote Dick, "and by the time the recipient's hands and nose are reached, levels drop to zero or nearly so."

"These early studies led us to believe that cold viruses did not survive on surfaces and that transmission had to be directly from hand-to-hand, and from there to nose or eye," says Birgit Winther. But no longer. With new, more sensitive technology for detecting viruses, Winther and others have found cold viruses surviving on a variety of different surfaces for long periods of time. Indeed, she has made a career of studying cold-virus transmission by way of hands and surfaces. And like Lovelock, she is deeply suspect of sneezing and breathing as conveyors of colds.

There is little evidence that coughs and sneezes actually produce an aerosol that spreads infection, says Winther. "With a sneeze, you feel a tickle in the nose, then there's a high-pressure expelling of air, along with secretions from a pool at the front of the mouth—not the nose," she says. And since saliva harbors little or no cold virus, aerosolized saliva initiated by a sneeze is unlikely to spread infection. In fact, when investigators sampled air for virus in a room that housed volunteers heavy with cold, they found no virus even though 82 percent of the air was sampled. Moreover, when volunteers coughed or sneezed directly onto a surface designed for virus detection, the researchers recovered virus from only 2 out of 25 sneezes.

Winther became convinced that colds were not spread easily through the air when she was a student working on a six-week cold study in a lab in Copenhagen. "We were 4 people in a small room," she recalls, "and we had 60 subjects, all of them with really severe colds from different kinds of cold viruses. You could hear them blowing their noses in the hall before they came in, and then they spent a long time in this little room with us. It was terrible. The room was humid with mucus, really disgusting." She and her collaborators were careful not to touch their faces while working with the sick volunteers. "Still, I fully expected all of us to come down with a cold," she says. "To our complete surprise, none of us did. It seemed absolutely unbelievable at the time. But now we understand that you have to be really, really close to someone to be infected by aerosols; we more often catch the virus with our hands."

To seal the theory of hand transmission, Jack Gwaltney Jr. and his team set out to interrupt the hand-to-nose chain of viral spread in a natural setting by treating mothers' hands with iodine. Solutions containing iodine had been found to be effective in keeping hands sterile for up to four hours. Gwaltney studied 50 families. Half of the mothers in the families used iodine to treat their hands on a regular basis when a family member came down with a cold. A control group of mothers treated their hands with a solution of brown food dye. The iodine reduced colds by 40 to 50 percent, says Gwaltney, and it reduced rhinovirus infection by 90 percent. (Unfortunately, the element's capacity for colorful staining has prevented its development as a viable hand treatment.)

Since then, Winther and her colleagues have discovered that rhinoviruses and other pathogens are adept at hopscotching to a new host by way of objects and surfaces such as Lovelock's playing cards and dinner dishes. It's true that there's a big drop-off of recoverable virus from a surface once it's dried (around 90 percent)—after all, a virus is an obligate parasite that depends on a host. However, what remains, the residual virus, can endure for surprisingly long periods of time. And as we know, it takes only one particle to infect. In the early 1980s, Jack Gwaltney Jr. and Owen Hendley discovered that more than half of people who handled coffee cup handles and other objects contaminated with rhinovirus caught colds. Another study, which used a bacteriophage—a virus that infects bacteria—as a marker, found that virus from an inoculated doorknob was transferred to 14 successive people who touched the knob and thence to an additional 6 people through handshakes.

"Transfer of viruses by way of surfaces may be inefficient," says Hendley, "but it's highly effective. Rhinoviruses may be on so many different damned surfaces that this is part and parcel of the way they get around."

Winther, Hendley, and their colleagues are continuing to sleuth the viral trek from nose to surface to fingertip in various settings. They have shown that if virus is left on a light switch at a hotel, and someone comes and flicks on that light switch an hour later or the next day, the virus will transfer. And if a toy in a doctor's office has been handled by a child with a cold, the next kid may well take the virus home, along with his "good patient" sticker.

There is new ammunition on the airborne front as well. One recent small study suggested that simple breathing might in fact generate virus-laden aerosols. Australian researchers asked nine patients with cold symptoms to wear special masks placed closely over nose and mouth while they read aloud for 20 minutes, breathed quietly for 20 minutes, and coughed 20 times. The masks captured rhinovirus in six patients, including three during simple breathing. But critics say it isn't clear whether the contamination was actually a result of aerosolization or just close contact with the mask, and there were no follow-up studies to see whether infection might spread by this route.

Despite more than 70 years of research, the precise paths cold viruses take to inflict their misery remain controversial. Both airborne and pedestrian routes undoubtedly play a part in our infection. "It probably depends on which cold virus you're exposed to," explains Ron Turner. "Colds caused by the influenza virus, for instance, may spread through small-particle aerosol. Airborne transmission of rhinovirus infection is also possible, but only with prolonged and close exposure. For most colds," says Turner, "it's probably direct contact."

So much for the how of catching cold. What about the where?

Not long ago, Charles Gerba, a microbiologist at the University of Arizona, sought to identify public areas where risk of exposure to all sorts of pathogens might be greatest. Gerba is a man obsessed with the germs that lurk in our daily lives. A professor of environmental microbiology, he has for the last two decades or so focused his beam on everyday hangouts for viruses and bacteria. He once invented what he calls a "commodograph" to measure the aerosol of droplets emitted with each flush from a toilet bowl. After an investigation revealed the presence of *E. coli* in laundry machines, including his own, he started running an empty load with bleach to "mouthwash" the machine.

In 2005, Gerba and his team reported trawling more than 1,000 public surfaces in four U.S. cities, from shopping centers, day-care facilities, offices, airports, movie theaters, restaurants, and other public locations, looking for biochemical markers of substances that would carry pathogens—blood, saliva, feces, urine, mucus, etc. They found that surfaces from children's playground equipment and day-care centers were the most contaminated—perhaps not shocking, but distressing nonetheless. When Gerba's team members used an invisible fluorescent resin to artificially contaminate surfaces, they revealed that 86 percent of people who touched the surfaces carried away the tracer. Eighty percent transferred it to their personal belongings or took it home hours later. Biggest offenders were children's playground equipment and bus rails and armrests, followed by shopping cart handles, chair armrests, vending machine buttons, and escalator handrails.

Gerba and other researchers more tightly focused on the whereabouts of cold viruses have journeyed into hotels, doctors' offices, child-care facilities, and people's homes to parse where they hang out. So what are the hot havens for cold viruses?

*   *   *

The Doctor's Office. If you have small children, you probably suspect as much: toys in pediatric waiting rooms almost certainly harbor cold viruses. Dr. Diane Pappas and her team at the University of Virginia used DNA sampling to test toys in three locations in pediatricians' offices in Fairfax, Virginia: a sick-child waiting room, a well-child waiting room, and a bag of new toys offered to reward little patients after their doctor visits. Some 17 percent of the toys in the waiting room for well children were contaminated; 20 percent of those in the room for sick children were buggy. The bag of new toy "rewards" was the worst, with some 30 percent of the toys carrying remnants of viruses. What's more, says Pappas, cleaning the toys according to office protocol with disinfectants only minimally decreased the presence of viral remnants, from 40 percent to 26 percent.

The (Jungle) Gym. Children's playground equipment is the germiest of surfaces. But cold bugs catch rides not just on jungle gyms and swings. When researchers looked for pathogens at two fitness centers in a military community in Hawaii, they found the presence of viruses (primarily rhinoviruses) on 63 percent of hand-contact surfaces. Especially contaminated were barbells, dumbbells, and weight plates, as well as grips for bicycles and stair-climbers.

The Elevator and Other Public Transportation. In Gerba's four-city study, bus rails and armrests were second only to playground equipment in contamination. As for elevators: I have a friend who works on the 17th floor of an office building in downtown Manhattan. Every morning she avoids the elevator and instead takes the stairs up to her office. Though she's aware of the health benefits of stair-climbing, it's not the exercise she craves. And while the crowding is considerable in the lift, it's not the claustrophobia factor that drives her to the stairwell. Rather, she sees the elevator as a virus's way of gaining perpendicular passage. She may have a point. Some experts suspect that the SARS epidemic spread when a professor from China, sick with the virus, stayed for a single night in room 911 on the ninth floor of Hong Kong's Metropole Hotel. By touching an elevator button, he may have unwittingly spread the disease to fellow guests. All 16 people who contracted SARS had stayed on the ninth floor or had a connection to it and would have been pressing that ninth-floor elevator button. Over the next few days, those 16 hotel guests spread the virus far and wide, to some 30 countries.

The Bank or Anywhere You Handle Cash. Scientists in Switzerland recently demonstrated that viruses survive on banknotes—and presumably dollar bills—for weeks. The team dripped a blend of flu viruses and human nasal mucus on the notes, left them at room temperature for varying periods of time, and then tested them for live virus. The researchers found that the dry viruses stayed viable for three days—and when they were mixed with the mucus, for more than two weeks. Whether viruses stuck on a dollar bill remain infectious depends on the number of particles attached and whether the bill stays wet enough to prevent their demise through drying. The chances of getting infected from handling money may also be a matter of the kind of contact you have with your bills—touch alone or something more intimate; say, the sort of "hoovering" that goes on when people snort drugs from bills, providing the virus with an expressway to the respiratory passages. Influenza viruses tend to survive longer on surfaces than most kinds of cold viruses, so if it's any comfort, there may be less risk of succumbing to their breed of snuffles from this sort of snort.

*   *   *

The Office. Though most colds are picked up not at the office but at home, it's still prudent to beware all routes of workplace spread.

Not long ago, a team of Boston scientists curious about the link between the stale air in offices and the incidence of colds decided to look at the rate of respiratory infections in office buildings with little outdoor ventilation. Studies during the Gulf War had shown that colds were more frequent among troops housed in air-conditioned barracks compared with those housed in tents. The Boston team tested the air filters in three poorly ventilated area office buildings and collected mucus samples from workers who complained of colds. They found airborne respiratory virus in 32 percent of the sample filters. The team also found a close genetic match between the rhinovirus in an air sample and the bug taken from a nasal mucus sample of a building occupant sick with a cold. The scientists suspect the sick office worker expelled this particular strain of rhinovirus, or else it was part of a chain of infection present in the building. The good news is that the filters caught at least some of the bugs; the bad news is that they were there in the first place.

Charles Gerba's 2002 study using fluorescent resin tracers on office surfaces turned up some unsettling news about the general presence of pathogens in offices. Resin from a faucet and an exit doorknob in an office bathroom hitched its way onto employees' hands, faces, phones, and hair. From a community phone, it migrated to pens, doorknobs, keyboards, and drinking cups; and from a copy machine button to documents, computers, and more hands and faces. Gerba also found that the average office desk—what he dubs a "laptop of luxury" for bacteria—has some 20,000 "coworkers" per square inch, around 400 times more bacteria than a toilet seat. Keyboards and the "enter" and "send" buttons on fax machines are likewise germ headquarters. Though women's offices often look cleaner, they typically harbor almost three times the number of bacteria as men's (in part because women tend to eat more healthy, biodegradable food at their desks). However, men's wallets are four times germier than women's purses. Germiest jobs are teacher, accountant, banker, radio DJ, doctor, TV producer, consultant, publicist, and lawyer.

As for viruses in the workplace, Gerba coordinated a study of offices in five cities to detect the presence of human parainfluenza 1 virus, a not uncommon cause of the common cold and other respiratory infections. More than 300 samples were collected from offices, cubicles, and conference rooms in New York, Atlanta, Chicago, Tucson, and San Francisco. The high-touch, high-contact areas were rife with virus: 47 percent of desktops, 46 percent of computer mice, and 45 percent of telephones. Tucson was the least virus-riddled city and New York the most, with half of its surfaces testing positive for the virus.

The point is this: infected office workers can leave a microbial trail on nearly everything they touch. According to Gerba, a person with a cold coats about 30 percent of a room's surfaces with viruses.

Day-Care Centers and Schools. "Unlike the old days, when we had our young children playing outside much of the day, now we concentrate them in little spaces," says Birgit Winther—"optimal circumstances for spreading viruses." While many kids with colds stay home from school (the average schoolchild takes 11 days off for colds each year), others hop on the bus anyway. It's now common knowledge that epidemics of colds start up with the start of school in late summer and early fall. "Some 17 days after children return to school, we see a peak in occurrence of respiratory infections three to four times the background rate," notes Sebastian Johnston of Imperial College London. "People go on vacation, come home with viruses, and the schoolchildren share them with all their friends." According to the Centers for Disease Control and Prevention, there are more than 52 million cases of the common cold each year among Americans under the age of 17.

In a study of the occurrence of viruses on elementary school classroom surfaces in 2009, Gerba found that half of the surfaces tested positive for virus. Frequently used fomites were the most contaminated: desktops, faucet handles, paper towel dispensers, and entrance doorknobs. (Teachers' desks are also germ havens, Gerba discovered in a previous study, harboring up to 20 times more microbes per square inch compared with desks of people in other professions—the reason my sister, a special education teacher in Maryland, slathers her desk with cleanser and washes her hands some 30 times a day.)

Studying virus transmission in a school or child-care facility is tricky. No scientist wants to plant real bugs for kids to pick up, so one enterprising group of scientists came up with a safe way of studying virus transmission in child-care facilities. They used a fragment of a plant virus, the cauliflower mosaic virus, as a surrogate marker to mimic a real human viral pathogen and smeared it onto toy balls; then they introduced the toy balls into several child-care settings. Within just a few hours of handling, the viral DNA on the toy balls had spread—to other, unsmeared balls, to the hands of the children and caregivers, to benches and boxes touched frequently by the children. Although the smeared balls were removed after a day, the viral DNA continued circulating in the facilities for as long as two weeks and showed up in the children's homes, on the hands of family members, and on several surfaces, including high chairs, toys, cribs, and bathtub rims.

*   *   *

The Home. Unfortunately, when children get colds at school or day care, they usually bring them home. Indeed, the presence of infants or children in a household doubles the cold rate for the adults living there. "If you have kids, chances are good that you'll get infected," says Ron Turner. "Our children transmit viruses efficiently because of the way we interact with them. We love them, so we wipe their noses."

But even households without kids are hardly bug-free. In sleuthing germs in 15 homes, Gerba discovered that the cleanest spot in the house—at least where bacteria are concerned—was the toilet seat; the dirtiest, the sponge or drain. "The cutting board was very bad," he writes. "There are 200 times more faecal coliforms [bacteria] on a cutting board than a toilet seat. From these data it would appear that the safest place to make a salad in the home seems to be on the top of the toilet seat."

In 2008 Winther's team looked specifically for rhinoviruses in the homes of people with colds. The team asked 30 cold-ridden adults to indicate 10 spots in their houses that they had touched in the past 18 hours, then tested the spots for the genetic fingerprints of the viruses. Sixty-seven of the 160 surfaces tested positive for rhinovirus. The genetic fingerprinting may have yielded some false positives. Nonetheless, says Winther, "surfaces in the home that are commonly touched by people are far more important than we ever imagined in the spread of colds."

To follow up, the team later deliberately contaminated commonly touched surfaces with the subjects' mucus and asked them to turn on the lights, answer the phone, and do other kinds of daily activities to see whether the virus on the object would stick to their fingers. After 1 hour, the virus fused to fingertip close to 90 percent of the time; after 24 hours, it had dropped only to 70 percent; and after 48 hours, to 53 percent. So even a full two days after the mucus was smeared, participants got the virus on their fingertips more than half the time.

Cold viruses may also lurk in less obvious spots. The tucks and folds of clothing, for instance—especially hankies and the shirtsleeves of children. "I never realized how risky doing laundry was," says Gerba. "It may be one of the major transfer points in the home for pathogenic microorganisms....Anyone transferring a load of underwear [from washer to dryer], for example, will get *E. coli* on their hands." Washing eliminates 99 percent of the bacteria, but if there are a million to begin with, that leaves some 10,000. And viruses are even harder to wash out of fabric than bacteria. "So laundry is a hazardous activity in the home," notes Gerba, "particularly if that home includes an ill individual or a small child: all those children's underwear and diapers, and soiled handkerchiefs when somebody has a cold."

The Hotel. In 2007, Birgit Winther and Owen Hendley conducted their infamous hotel study showing that adults infected with rhinovirus left viral RNA on a third of the 150 or so objects and surfaces they touched in their hotel rooms in the course of normal daily activities. Most contaminated were door handles and pens. A close second were light switches, faucets, TV remotes, and telephones—all surfaces rarely scoured by cleaning crews. And here's the big disenchantment to those of us checking in to a "clean" hotel room: The RNA from the viruses remained on these surfaces for as long as 18 hours. The researchers found that 1 hour after contamination, rhinovirus RNA transferred from surfaces to fingertips in 18 out of 30 trials, and 18 hours after contamination, in 10 out of 30 trials. "The next time you stay in a hotel," says Hendley, "you may wonder how meticulous the cleanup crew was with their work."

The Plane. Most of us don't put off our scheduled flights because we have a cold—which means that we seal ourselves (and our viruses) into a small, enclosed space in close proximity to hundreds of fellow travelers, with what would seem to be predictable results.

One hot day in July 2008, three minutes before my plane was scheduled to take off from Charlottesville en route to Washington, D.C., the pilot, Captain Scott, popped out of the cabin and announced to his passengers that he wanted to high-five each of us before he took off, he said, "just to be sure that I make a safe landing. It's my little superstition; I never fly without my high fives." A twitter of disbelief traversed the rows. One humorless man in the seat across the aisle from me glared at Scott with annoyance and kept his hands pinned to his sides. "Can we please just take off? Captain? Sir?" But Scott insisted, cajoling and teasing until the man finally held out a pinky for the pilot to flick so that he would get on with his task. With the research on hand-to-hand transmission of colds fresh in my mind, my foremost thought was how happy I was to be seated in the first row. My only exposure would come from Scott and my reluctant partner across the aisle, both of whom looked healthy. So I raised my palm obligingly, and Captain Scott, grinning broadly, made his way to the rear of the plane, hand-slapping each and every passenger. We took off without further incident. Thirty minutes later, however—high fives notwithstanding—we had a singularly rough landing. While taxiing to the gate, I asked the flight attendant if the captain completed this strange ritual before every flight. "Yes," she said in a low voice. "And it seems a little unprofessional to me." She continued in a whisper, "I think it makes the passengers nervous."

Yes, and probably more apt to leave with a sneeze. But even without a crazy pilot to spread germs, is flying a cold hazard? Do the special circumstances of air travel—the general stress, the confined space, the close and prolonged exposure to some 400 other passengers (especially during long-haul flights)—all conspire to boost our chances of leaving a jet with more than just our carry-on?

One recent study seemed to suggest so. When scientists from the University of California surveyed more than 1,000 passengers flying between San Francisco and Denver, they found that 20 percent reported experiencing cold symptoms within a week of flying. That's a very high rate of incidence, roughly four times the risk than if they'd stayed at home.

One popular theory fingers cabin ventilation systems as the culprit in the spread of disease on airplanes, particularly those that recirculate air. The importance of a well-function-ing cabin ventilation system in preventing the spread of flu and other commonly airborne bugs was made clear by a case in 1979, when an Alaskan passenger jet suffered engine failure during takeoff. The plane sat on the ground for three hours while the engine was repaired, and the cabin ventilation sys-tem was turned off. One passenger developed symptoms of flu. Within three days, 72 percent of the passengers and 40 percent of the crew had come down with the flu. Because of this case, it's now recommended that aircraft ventilation be supplied for ground delays of more than a half hour.

Recirculating ventilation systems have long been under suspicion as the perpetrators of illness in air travel. Certainly, if cold viruses travel by aerosol, one would think that this new strategy of recirculating air in planes would be a fine mode of travel for frequent-flier bugs in search of fresh hosts. In the past, commercial planes used 100 percent fresh air, cooled by engines in an energy-consuming way. Newer planes, built since the 1980s, are designed to recirculate about half of cabin air, reducing the engine's work and thereby boosting fuel efficiency. Most of the old fresh-air model planes are being retired, but many are still in use on that California-to-Colorado route studied by the University of California team. The two types of air systems suggested to the team a natural experiment: comparing rates of cold symptoms reported by the passengers flying between San Francisco and Denver after travel in one type of plane or the other. It turned out that there was little difference. A week after flying, one in five passengers in both kinds of planes suffered respiratory symptoms.

In truth, the filters used in these recirculation systems are similar to those used in hospital operating theaters and sterile wards and are highly effective at removing some 99.9 percent of bacteria and viruses from cabin air. The air is completely exchanged at least 20 times per hour, compared with 12 air exchanges per hour in most office buildings and only 5 per hour in most homes. In short, the resulting air quality generally exceeds that found in most enclosed spaces on terra firma.

The offender may not be recirculation but the air itself, whether fresh or recirculated—at least according to Martin Hocking of the University of Victoria in Canada. In Hocking's view, the issue is humidity, or the lack thereof. Because the air at high altitudes is practically devoid of moisture, the typical humidity in aircraft cabins for flights longer than an hour is below 10 percent for most of the journey, and for longer journeys may drop to less than 5 percent. Hocking suspects that the dry air lowers our resistance to respiratory infections. Some experiments have shown that when air is dry, the thin layer of mucus in our nose and throat that traps viruses and moves them to the stomach for destruction by acids ceases to function well. Not everyone buys this idea. Some experts hold that our ability to clear our mucus isn't hampered by dry conditions. In any case, you would think boosting the humidity in aircraft air wouldn't be rocket science. But when British Airways tried to humidify a Boeing 747 aircraft in the 1980s, the air conditioner sprayed out tiny white pellets along with the air supply, showering the interior (and especially the flight deck) with fake snow. If you're concerned about nasal drying, it may be safer to carry your own humidity in the form of a nasal saline spray.

Jack Gwaltney Jr. isn't so sure those passengers in the University of California survey actually had colds. They were never tested for the presence of viruses, so there's a good possibility they just had respiratory symptoms that they reported as colds. He doesn't believe there's a higher incidence of colds in people who fly. But conditions inside the cabin may indeed promote symptoms that feel like a cold—stuffy or runny nose. Airborne infections like flu are another matter, says Gwaltney. "If you're on a plane with a lady down with the flu, there's a very good chance you'll get sick, too."

Chapter 3

THE BUGS

A microbe is so very small
You cannot make him out at all.

JOSEPH HILAIRE PIERRE RENÉ BELLOC

Cold viruses may be among the world's most successful human pathogens, causing more infections than any other germ, but as Belloc says, they're not much to look at.

"A typical cold virus such as a rhinovirus is so small that you can't see it—even with a powerful standard electron microscope," says Birgit Winther. "It just looks like dots of dirt." With only an ordinary light microscope, a child can see the satisfying plump wiggle of any reputable bacterium. But cold viruses are so vanishingly small at 20 nanometers across that they can barely be seen at the 100,000× magnification of a powerful electron microscope. Things this tiny are nearly as hard to fathom as the very, very large, even if you tell me that 50,000 of them would fit side by side in the space of a millimeter or 2,400 in the width of a hair. Or put otherwise: if we enlarged the world like *Alice in Wonderland*, blowing up one rhinovirus particle to, say, the size of a golf ball, in comparison your Bunyan-like body, sprawled across the United States, would run from sea to sea.

"Only when you stain them does the pattern of their presence emerge," explains Winther. In fact, crystallographers can make a rhinovirus look quite elegant, with an icosahedral, or twenty-sided, symmetrical structure. If you zoomed in even closer, you might see a miniature terrain like a moonscape, with numerous little canyons. But these views are completely artificial, visual tricks. A cold virus is less like an organism and more like a very simple chemistry set: a single strand of genetic material, in this case RNA, tightly coiled inside a rigid protein capsule called a capsid. It is, as virologist Peter Medawar once described all viruses, just a bit of "bad news wrapped in a protein coat." Nonetheless it braves the outside world to cause each of us some 24,000 hours of congestive misery over a lifetime.

You can understand how hard it would be for scholars of the past to imagine that something so small it couldn't be seen might wreak such havoc. The ancients saw colds as the product of that vague foggy thing, the miasma, or as an imbalance of bodily "humors." In fact, the word *catarrh*, still used in some circles, derives from Hippocrates' use of *katarrhous*, the "flowing down" of humors from the head. The brain, preternaturally affected by cold, produced an excess of phlegm, which would leak out through the small holes in the floor of the skull and run out of the nose (that is, if it didn't leak into joints and cause rheumatism).

"Obstructed perspiration" is how William Buchan delicately referred to a snotty nose in his *Domestic Medicine* of 1772. As for cause, Buchan pointed an accusatory finger at wet clothes, wet feet ("which often occasion fatal diseases"), night air (especially evening dews, the effects of which, though "gradual and imperceptible," are "not the less to be dreaded"), damp beds, damp houses, and sudden transitions from heat to cold. "Indeed, if the human body could be kept constantly in an uniform degree of warmth," he wrote, "such a thing as catching cold would be impossible."

And yet, as early as the 1770s, the prescient Benjamin Franklin suspected something besides temperature was at work here. Always ahead of his time, Franklin dismissed cold and dampness as the culprits in the common cold. "Travelling in our severe Winters, I have suffered Cold sometimes to an Extremity only short of Freezing," he wrote in 1773, "but this did not make me *catch Cold.*" As for moisture: "I have been in the River every Evening two or three Hours for a Fortnight... when one would suppose I might imbibe enough of it to take Cold if Humidity could give it; but no such Effect followed." Instead, Franklin suspected that the root cause was an agent transmitted from person to person. "People often catch Cold from one another when shut up together in small close Rooms, Coaches, &c." he wrote, "and when sitting near and conversing so as to breathe in each others Transpiration."

By the mid-1800s the great microbe hunters, Louis Pasteur in Paris and Robert Koch in Berlin, had peered into their microscopes and shown that there were indeed minute organisms capable of causing infectious disease. It was a small logical step to conclude that the common cold might be caused by one of these newfound "pus-producing bacteria"—and only a matter of time before researchers probing the noses of cold sufferers uncovered what they believed to be two culprits: *Micrococcus catarrhalis* and *Bacillus rhinitis.* But it soon surfaced that the bacterial bugs were falsely accused. They turned up in the noses and throats of healthy people, too, in greater numbers than in the cold-stricken.

At the start of World War I, a researcher working in Leipzig first demonstrated that the nasal flow from someone sick with a cold was capable of producing fresh colds in another person. Walter Kruse took nasal secretions from a hapless assistant who suffered a bad head cold and passed them through a ceramic filter that captured bacteria. When he put a few drops of the resulting clear filtrate into the noses of 12 volunteers, 4 of them reported that they developed colds. Kruse concluded that the infectious cause of the common cold was something smaller than a bacterium, a "filterable virus" he called *Aphanozoum coryzae*. But it was not until 1930 that a group of affable young chimpanzees helped to settle the matter.

The idea of employing chimps as experimental cold subjects was the brainchild of Alphonse Dochez (pronounced Dokay), a physician at Columbia University. Dochez understood that studying the cause of the common cold in humans was tricky: first, because of the difficulty of quarantining human subjects, so as to be sure the colds they caught were from the nose drops they were given rather than from something they picked up while they were out and about; and second, because of the willingness of subjects to oblige the researchers by reporting imagined colds. As cold researcher George Gee Jackson once said, "Man as a species for experimental study is probably the most cantankerous, unreliable, neurotic, and variable that could be chosen." The more reliable alternative of chimps occurred to Dochez after he learned from zoo curators that the primates readily caught colds from their human keepers; here were subjects far less likely to be "self-convinced" of infection.

A chimp with a cold looks a lot like a sick child, Dochez observed, with thick, "glairy" snot in the nostrils, a thin stream of mucus running over the upper lip, drooping eyes, stuffiness, difficulty breathing, and general mopiness and lassitude. Dochez found that by inoculating the chimps' noses with filtered, bacteria-free nasal washings from a sick human, he could readily give them a cold. Within 24 hours, their noses were running, they were sneezing, and their eyes looked puffy. He subsequently performed his experiment on humans and concluded that "the active agent present in these filtrates, by means of which we have been able to transmit colds, is a true submicroscopic virus."

This was a big breakthrough. But the nature of the viral agent remained a mystery. To identify a virus, you have to be able to isolate it and grow it. Doing so with the cold virus turned out to be devilishly difficult, like stalking a wild animal, as one researcher described it. Sir Christopher Andrewes, a British virologist familiar with Dochez's work, launched a fresh attack on the problem in the early 1930s. With funds in short supply, he could not afford chimpanzees, so he recruited medical students from the local St. Bartholomew's Hospital—because, he said, "the next best thing to a chimpanzee is a Bart's student." An "unsatisfactory" substitute, he added, but "the only animals available."

A bevy of mobile medical students, however, is not exactly the sort of tightly controlled arrangement suited to isolating a cold virus. Ideally, volunteers themselves should be isolated so that researchers can be sure any colds they suffer result from the viral inoculations they receive and not from a "wild cold" caught from outside contacts. So in 1946 Andrewes opened the Common Cold Unit, what would become the leading research center on cold viruses for almost four decades.

The CCU, as it was known, occupied the old Harvard Hospital, a cluster of structures situated on a windswept hilltop just outside Salisbury in southern England, a few miles from the ancient stone pillars of Stonehenge and not far from Porton Down, the government research laboratory for chemical and biological defense. Built by Americans in 1941 to house victims of cholera, typhoid, and other epidemics they expected might result from the crowding in shelters during wartime bombing, the hospital was a series of interconnected camouflaged huts 120 feet long and detached to minimize the risk of cross-infection and destruction from German attack. The epidemics never materialized, and the hospital sat empty until it drew Andrewes's eye. You can see from old photographs that the buildings themselves had the look of a POW camp, but the site was "delightfully light and airy," as Andrewes described it, "with magnificent views across to chalk downs." In Andrewes's mind, it was the perfect setup to house his human guinea pigs.

During the several decades thereafter, some 20,000 volunteers, up to 30 at a time (the predecessors of my own little study group at UVA), were invited to spend 10 days as experimental subjects in the CCU's small, sparsely furnished flats. The unit paid the volunteers' travel expenses, gave them free lodging and food, and even provided a little pocket money. In return, the volunteers submitted to experiments and around a 40 percent chance of catching a cold.

The CCU quickly won notoriety in Britain as a kind of eccentric and charming mix of high-tech virology laboratory and old-fashioned British holiday camp where doctors in white lab coats tested old wives' tales about colds. There was no shortage of applicants, and many volunteers so relished the experience they got "hooked on the virus habit," as one newspaper put it, and made return visits again and again. One couple, parents to six children, came regularly to escape their brood. The record went to two volunteers who attended 15 times. Applicants turned up from other countries, including an American boxer who asked only that arrangements be made for a visit to the queen and a contest with the leading British heavyweight. The lab even found its way into Iris

Murdoch's novel *Under the Net*: "It was through the common cold that I first met Hugo," says the novel's restless and rebellious hero Jake Donaghue. "This was in a period when I was particularly short of cash, and things went very ill indeed with me until I discovered an incredibly charitable arrangement whereby I could get free board and lodging in exchange for being a guinea pig in a cold cure experiment."

Today the sole memorial to the CCU is a small plaque at the site of a housing development. But the volunteers are still circulating. Angela Greenslade and Janet Wilson-Ward met when they were matched as roommates at the CCU in 1972. Solitary confinement for ten days would be unwelcome to most people, as Andrewes put it, so volunteers were normally paired up. Apparently the staff excelled at matching compatible strangers. In 2008, I joined Angela and Janet for lunch at a restaurant in Covent Garden while they were in London celebrating Janet's 60th birthday, more than 35 years after their shared cold adventure. Janet, now a law professor at the University of Bath, had learned about the CCU from an ad in an alternative newspaper when she was a law student and went there looking for a free holiday and some quiet study time. She found that as well as a lifelong friend. Angela, who works at Sotheby's, describes her three "holidays" at the CCU as glorious, completely happy experiences. "I've never laughed so much in my life," she told me. "It was heaven." The volunteers had hot meals delivered to them in thermos containers by staff wearing masks, free lager, and the use of the library and sports facilities. They were even provided with Wellington boots to walk the acres of chalk grasslands. "It felt like a school holiday," Angela said, "without the teachers." A cold was small price to pay.

When they arrived, the volunteers were assigned to their flats, then given a talk by staff outlining the various rules.

Angela says that she chose this moment to ask the doctors, only half-jokingly, whether there was any link between the CCU and the nearby defense laboratory, Porton Down. It was a legitimate question. In the 50 years between 1939 and 1989, Porton Down was the site of various trials involving chemical and biological research on thousands of volunteer servicemen attracted to the research program by the prospect of a weekend pass and 15 shillings. Some of the volunteers say they were told they would be participating in research aimed at finding a cure for the common cold and instead were given hallucinogens, mustard gas, sarin, and other nerve agents. In 1953 Ronald Maddison, a 20-year-old Air Force engineer whose family said he was under the impression he was volunteering to help with cold research, was isolated in a chamber and exposed to sarin dripped onto a piece of material wrapping his arm. He died an hour later. More than half a century after the experiments, the British secret intelligence body MI6 made out-of-court settlements with some of the ex-servicemen who participated in the program, though it admitted no liability or wrongdoing.

Angela says that a somewhat humorless CCU doctor assured her and her fellow volunteers that there was no link between this cold research and Porton. He then went on to instruct them all in stern terms to keep a distance of 30 feet from every other person except their roommate and protected staff members. The distance was somewhat arbitrary, but the purpose was to keep the volunteers at a safe remove from other people who might transmit a "private enterprise" cold virus. "If you met another person when you were out walking you had to cover your face," Janet said. "There was a Gypsy camp nearby, and the staff had to explain to them that volunteers who saw them and suddenly put their hands or scarves over their faces weren't being rude."

Some volunteers tested the in-house distance rules. A couple of days after checking in to the CCU, Angela confided, she and Janet were settling down for the night and watching TV in their flat when there was a tap on the window. It was a boy Angela had met at the pep-talk session. "I shrieked when I saw it was him as I had giant hair curlers in and cream all over my face," she recalls with a blush. "I rushed out of sight to take the curlers out and cream off and then I joined him for bit of innocent necking outside the hut. I was worried that someone might see us and send us home for breaking the rules of isolation, so I soon sent him on his merry way. But it certainly added to the fun, drama, and the sheer surreal quality of our stay there." Other CCU romances flourished despite the distance rule. One guitar-playing volunteer who came to the unit nine times recalls that on one visit he fell for an oboist and played duets with her at 30 feet. Some courtships even blossomed into marriage.

After their pep talk, the volunteers were isolated for two days and monitored to see if they developed a cold. If they did, it meant they had been exposed to a wild-type cold virus before they arrived, and they were sent home. On the third day of isolation, the remaining volunteers were given the cold virus challenge. "We had to lie down with our heads tilted back while scientists dressed in masks and gowns dripped fluid in our noses," Janet recalls. "It was bizarre and comical, like being in a film." (I know the feeling.) The fluid was either placebo—a plain saline solution—or contained live cold virus derived from nasal washings provided by staff members or other volunteers with colds. Not even the scientists knew which volunteers got which solution until after the study. Nowadays this so-called double-blind, placebo-controlled approach is standard in clinical trials, but in the early experiments at the CCU, it was quite an innovation.

Over the next five days the volunteers were watched for symptoms. Every morning they were visited by a staff physician who felt their glands and measured their breathing. Later, someone would come by to collect the day's used tissues, which the volunteers collected and stored in sealed in plastic bags. On her second visit Janet caught a lulu of a cold and used 80 tissues a day for three days. The daily record was 165. But just counting tissues wasn't a sufficient index of cold severity, observed Andrewes. Some volunteers would toss a tissue after dabbing the nose once; others would use one tissue repeatedly until it was a "soggy mess" or had "disintegrated into shreds." Better to weigh the bags, then subtract the weight of the tissue and bag and voilà: the weight of fluid that had run from the nose as a quantifiable measurement of cold severity—a standard that's still in use today in some cold studies.

In this way, the CCU investigated cold-related questions for close to 40 years, from how colds varied from season to season, to how close people needed to be to transfer illness; whether stress or personality was a factor in susceptibility; and the impact of large doses of orange juice on the progress of a cold.

Among Andrewes's earliest experiments, published in the early 1950s, was one he described as "rather harsh," designed to explore the ancient and nearly universal belief that chilling induces colds. He inoculated a group of volunteers with cold virus. Half of the group members were kept warm and comfortable; the other half took a hot bath, then stood about in a cool corridor scantily clad in wet bathing attire for half an hour "or as long as they could bear it," said Andrewes. Finally they were allowed to dress but had to wear wet socks for several hours. The chilled group felt miserable but didn't get any more colds than the warm group. "In not one instance did chilling alone produce a cold," wrote Andrewes, and in two out of three tests, chilling along with viral inoculation actually produced fewer colds than inoculation alone.

Meanwhile, in one desperate attempt after another, Andrewes and his colleagues at the CCU tried to grow cold viruses outside the human body to study them, first in eggs, then in human embryo cells, then in various animals, by inoculating them with cold washings from a human, but all without success. They tried to infect kittens, voles, squirrels (both gray and flying), ferrets, mice, rats, hamsters, rabbits, guinea pigs, hedgehogs, monkeys, baboons, a sooty mangabey, and more than one pig—much to the delight of the meat-starved postwar British staff, who got to dine on the failures. The researchers were forced to conclude that apart from chimpanzees, animals just didn't catch human colds. (Cats get awful colds but from cat cold viruses, not human ones.)

The best environment for growing the bug would seem to be the cells of the human nose, observed David Tyrrell, then a member of the CCU research team (and later its director). But nose cells had one distinct disadvantage—they're attached to the rest of the human. And alas, the viruses would not grow in an incubator set for the temperature of the human body. Then it dawned on Tyrrell that the temperature of the nasal passages, where cold viruses grow naturally, might be cooler than the rest of body. When he checked the temperature inside his own nose, he found it to be 91.4 degrees Fahrenheit rather than 97 or 98 degrees. Tyrrell figured out that cold viruses must thrive at these lower temperatures rather than the warmer climate of the blood and internal organs. When he reduced the temperatures of the incubator to 91.4 degrees, he successfully grew and cultured a bug, which later came to be christened as a rhinovirus for its favored nasal habitat.

The breakthrough came too late, however; it was two American physicians who simultaneously and independently won the rhinovirus isolation race. William Mogabgab first reported the discovery of a rhinovirus strain in 1956. While working at the Great Lakes Naval Training Station, the U.S. Navy's headquarters command for training in Chicago, Mogabgab had managed to isolate the virus from naval recruits with a mild respiratory illness.

At the same time, Winston Price, a public health specialist at Johns Hopkins University, discovered the rhinovirus quite by accident during a large outbreak of what he thought was flu. A group of nurses at Johns Hopkins came down with a bug that caused mild fever, cough, runny nose, and sore throat. Price collected throat and nasal washings from the sick nurses and then, when he realized they were getting no sicker, he suspected he had a cold virus. He grew the virus slowly in a solution of monkey kidney cells, horse serum, and beef embryo extract, and then isolated it. Price won public acclaim when he announced a year later that a vaccine made from the isolated virus was effective in preventing the cold. "The telephone by my bed kept ringing until 3 o'clock in the morning," he told one reporter. Newspapers all over the country wanted to know if this meant the end of the common cold. It didn't, of course. The inoculation was useful against only the one strain of cold virus. But if the vaccine didn't pan out, the techniques for isolating cold viruses certainly did, allowing a rash of discoveries of new strains over the ensuing decades.

We now know that colds are caused not by a single virus but by at least five unrelated families of viruses. More than half of these have been identified over the years by growing the viruses in culture. But it was a breakthrough in DNA technology that gave researchers the ability to identify new viruses quickly and easily. Polymerase chain reaction (PCR) is a technique that allows scientists to make millions of copies of a specific DNA sequence in just a couple of hours. With the help of PCR, scientists have discovered even more previously unknown cold viruses, among them the bocavirus (a kind of parvovirus), the human metapneumovirus (HMPV, first discovered in 2001, but which has likely been circulating in humans for at least 50 years), and many new strains of rhinovirus.

Until the 1990s, the insensitivity of viral detection and identification techniques led scientists to believe that rhinoviruses played a relatively minor role in disease. "But with the advent of better technology for identifying viral perpetrators of illness, we've discovered that rhinoviruses are major players in many serious illnesses," says Birgit Winther. With PCR-based methods, rhinoviruses that couldn't be detected by other means began popping up everywhere as perpetrators of—or at least participants in—attacks of asthma, otitis media (ear infections), and acute sinusitis. In 2007, a group of pediatricians from the University of Wisconsin found that more than half of rhinoviruses detected in seriously sick infants were previously unknown strains, including up to 50 that may represent a whole new group, the so-called group C. And it's likely that the viruses that cause as many as half of colds in adults haven't even been identified yet.

The enemy, it seems, is not the one but the many.

Cold viruses in the rhinovirus family are by far the most common, accounting for around half of all colds. The family is a veritable viral supergroup, with at least 100 genetically distinct strains that react to different antibodies. (Some scientists suspect the number of rhinovirus serotypes may be closer to 200.) In 2007, researchers announced that they had sequenced the genome of rhinoviruses, teasing apart some of their secrets. Having an abundance of strains is very clever of the rhinovirus family. Our immune systems are built to recognize antigens— little protein flags or markers on the surface of viruses, bacteria, and other invaders. When we have an encounter with a bug marked by a particular flag, the immune system builds a whole armament of antibodies earmarked for that flag. But those antibodies won't recognize other flags. The clever part is this: The different strains of rhinoviruses probably share lots of similar elements that could be constant flags for the immune system. However, each strain sports a different little decoy flag, which in essence distracts the immune system. It's a little like a bank robber who wears a mask with a long nose, explains Ron Turner. The nose is so distracting that witnesses can't remember what the robber's hair looks like. All rhinovirus strains may have blond hair, but each wears a different little nose mask, and the immune system, focusing only on the nose, can't recognize the bug as a familiar intruder. So when it comes to immunity, there's no cross-protection between the different rhinovirus strains.

Out there in the world of infections, then, there's something like a Cold Virus of the Month Club. The annual epidemic starts with a rash of rhinovirus infections in September, followed by a plethora of parainfluenza viruses in October and November. Winter sees a boost in respiratory syncytial viruses, human metapneumovirus, influenza, and coronaviruses. And then the rhinoviruses return, completing the cycle with a small wave of infections in March and April. Summertime is owned by enteroviruses.

The familiar seasonal outbreaks of colds are really the sum of minioutbreaks by a great number of different types of viruses spreading themselves about in similar fashion. Even a fairly small town may host as many as 80 different viral serotypes in a single cold season. (This "gang" mode of infection is in stark contrast to the serial style of the influenza virus—one flu virus generally replaces another so that only one or two influenza viruses circulate simultaneously.) In fact, researchers have found that within a single human family, more than

one strain of rhinovirus may be circulating—sibling bugs causing brother and sister the same miseries. Even an individual
person can carry more than one cold virus at a time, though
there's no reason to believe that the double dose results in a
more severe cold.

Different bugs tend to favor different habitats. Rhinoviruses prefer the snug nasopharynx; the parainfluenza virus
likes the voice box and the trachea; respiratory syncytial
viruses go for the small airways of the lung; and influenza
viruses favor the lung itself. Each bug can set off a spectrum
of symptoms, from minor cough and sneeze to a full-blown
flulike illness. For example, influenza viruses can cause simple
colds, while rhinoviruses can trigger symptoms like those seen
with the flu. Ron Turner suspects that the difference may come
down not just to host factors—age and susceptibility—but also
to the site of infection. An influenza virus that is inhaled by
aerosol and deposits itself in the large airways will cause typical flulike symptoms. But if it's delivered by direct contact into
the nose, it may elicit only mild cold symptoms.

In parsing the plethora of cold bugs, scientists have turned
up some strange discoveries. They had expected rhinoviruses
to look a lot like influenza viruses, but they better resemble
the poliovirus, sharing about half of the same genes. They're
not the major troublemakers polioviruses are because the proteins that coat them have lost their ability to survive in the
warm, acidic milieu of the gut and are generally happiest in
the cooler orifice of the nose. Human metapneumovirus originated in birds and may have jumped the species barrier around
two centuries ago. Respiratory syncytial virus, first isolated in
a chimp with a cold, causes mild colds in adults. But in children, this viral infection often develops into pneumonia or
bronchiolitis, especially in winter.

And here's a shocking new finding: some kinds of adenoviruses seem capable of triggering not just congestion but obesity. Three types of adenovirus normally spur only symptoms of the common cold, but in 20 percent of people, they may also affect the rate of fat-cell formation (playing a role in changing stem cells into fat cells to increase fat storage) so that those infected with the virus gain weight faster than noninfected people who eat the same amount of food. It's a discovery that—to my mind anyway—evokes nightmare scenarios of getting sneezed on in an elevator and emerging with the makings of both cold and corpulence.

Though these various cold bugs differ in their heritage and makeup, they all lead the same kind of borrowed life, sponging off human cells for their livelihood, and in the process, playing mischief with our lives. But is it fair to pin our miseries on the bugs themselves? Science suggests otherwise.

Chapter 4

THE HAVOC

Let us not look for our disease outside of ourselves;
it is planted in our entrails.

<small>SENECA</small>

You know the woes: First the stubborn little fist lodged in the pharynx that makes swallowing painful. Then the clogging congestion, the sneezing and free-flowing nose, the raw nostrils. Symptoms typically peak around the third day and ruin our hours for another three or four days, although they sometimes persist for longer, especially in children.

There may be more than 200 cold viruses, but once any cold bug launches an infection, the resulting spectrum of symptoms is pretty much the same. How can this be? It's not that the viruses are all so similar. The answer, we've learned lately, resides in the old Pogo line: "We have met the enemy, and he is us."

Until a couple of decades ago, science assumed that symptoms from any disease arose from the bugs themselves or from the toxins they produced. Cold viruses were no exception. After all, rhinoviruses killed cells in cell culture. "We all just assumed that when you had a terrible cold, your nose was falling apart inside," says Birgit Winther. A cold's miseries were thought to be the upshot of the cold virus's destruction of the innocent cells lining the nose—just as the miseries of flu arose from the flu virus's devastating effects on cells of the lower respiratory tract.

That was before Winther and her Danish colleagues thought to probe the nose in a most unusual way. At the time, Winther was a medical student studying at the University of Copenhagen with Niels Mygind, an expert in nasal biopsy-ing—a technique he used to show that spraying steroids in the nose reduces allergic symptoms. Mygind suggested to Winther that she look closely at the nature of the damage to the lining of the nose caused by the cold. So Winther and her fellow students set out to compare normal nose tissue with the injured tissue resulting from a cold. They took biopsies of nasal tissue in 56 people with severe natural colds. Two weeks later they biopsied the same group of people after they had recovered from their cold. Then the team did a blind evaluation of both sets of samples under a standard light microscope and also the powerful lens of a scanning electron microscope.

The result of all this nasal gazing? "We were shocked," says Winther. "We found absolutely no evidence of damage to the nasal lining in any of the samples. When I looked under a light microscope at the nasal samples from people in the second and third days of their colds, I did see an influx of polys [polymorphonuclear cells, a kind of white blood cell]. This coincided with the familiar onset of runny nose, sneezing, and other symptoms. But the actual nasal epithelial cells of people with colds and without colds all looked completely normal.

"This was very different from what we expected, and we thought, 'Hmm…what did we do wrong?' It took me quite a while before I finally accepted that what we found was right."

Elsewhere other evidence was emerging of the rhinoviruses' innocence. In the noses of those with infections, for instance, only an extremely small number of cells showed signs of replicating virus. "Some viruses such as influenza do direct damage to the body," says Jack Gwaltney Jr.; "they're very destructive to the respiratory epithelium." Others infect only a tiny number of epithelial cells lining the nasal passages and do very little harm. This is the case with rhinoviruses. "Rhinoviruses are not ripping up cells as we suspected," explains Gwaltney; "rather, they turn on processes in the body that under normal conditions are not active." Some of these so-called inflammatory processes help fend off or demolish viruses—but they also make us miserable.

So here was a blow to one of the nose's deepest secrets and the start of a new cold theory: cold symptoms do not result from the destructive effects of viruses after all but from the body's response to these intruders.

In other words, we make our own colds. In response to the presence of a virus, the body sets in motion an inflammatory cascade. It would require a large white board and several markers to diagram exactly what happens next. But in simple terms: The body's cells release a complex brew of chemicals called cytokines. These little hormonelike substances run all over the body, mediating and regulating our immune responses, mobilizing white blood cells to destroy pathogens. Some cytokines, such as interferon, attack viruses directly by inhibiting their replication inside our cells. Others (called proinflammatory cytokines) are like provocative emails, exciting immune activity. In response to the indignant messages, the body "inflames" its own cells and tissues, giving us a runny nose, cough, pain— all the building blocks of those troublesome cold symptoms. Thus our defense becomes our disease, making good on that old Pogo line.

In fact, you could create an artificial cold with no cold virus at all, says Gwaltney, just the cocktail of ingredients normally produced by the body in response to virus. The recipe would include a big squeeze of proinflammatory cytokines to rev up the immune system, among them a smidgeon of kinins to kindle sore throat, congestion, and runny nose; a pinch of prostaglandins to trigger cough; a hint of histamine to stimulate sneezing; and finally, for good measure, a dash of interleukins to foster lethargy.

In a real cold, it all starts when the virus makes its way to your pharynx and attaches to adenoidal cells there. In response, the cells make kinins, which stimulate nerve fibers, causing that sensation of dry scratchiness that augurs a cold. Later, the infection spreads forward, into your nose. The epithelial cells in the nose's moist mucosal lining become powerful little middlemen, kick-starting the body's mobilization of cytokines and white blood cells, and the cascade begins.

Eventually the inflammatory response leads to a full-fledged "adaptive" immune response, resulting in the production of antibodies that will protect you from the particular virus that started off the whole frenzy. Infection-fighting white blood cells known as T cells speed to the site from the bloodstream and lymph nodes and begin destroying the infected cells, along with their pirate viruses. On their arrival, the T cells release cytokines of their own, which mobilize so-called B cells. These make antibodies specifically directed against a particular cold virus. The antibodies don't actually fight the virus immediately but become useful in later encounters with it. The cytokines stimulate the B cells to multiply and make more antibodies. Finally, after several days, the viruses die off, and the immune cells retreat. What remains is a permanent memory of the infection, carried by antibodies and the B cells that made them. Run into this bug again, and your body will be ready to fight it off instantly, before it can cause infection.

When scientists peered into the body's cells in 2008 to see what was going on there in response to a cold virus, they discovered an astonishing amount of genetic activity. The team looked at each gene in the human genome—tens of thousands of genes tucked within each cell—to see if it made more or less of its normal gene product in people with colds as compared to healthy people. What they revealed was an immune system in serious overdrive. Forty-eight hours after infection, some 6,530 genes in the colds group showed changes in their expression. When the team classified the active genes by function, they found that many produced those proinflammatory cytokines, which play a role in chemotaxis, the process that recruits immune cells to the site of infection. Others made cytokines that calm the inflammatory response; still others made powerful antiviral compounds that directly help fend off cold and flu viruses.

In other words, the immune system is a little like an organic Internet—an enormously complex, interconnected communication system with many different kinds of cells and molecules that respond to germs in many different ways. The key to a healthy immune response to any infection is a delicate matter of balance or regulation of these different elements.

It's worth stepping back for a moment to parse this idea. Misunderstanding can lead to the wholesale swallowing of dubious claims by industry advertising that this cereal or that dietary supplement can fight colds by "boosting" the immune system. A recent example: Kellogg's effort in the midst of the swine flu epidemic to promote Cocoa Krispies as an "immune booster." In 2009, the company raised the percentage of four vitamins in the chocolaty, sweetened cereal from 10 percent to 25 percent of the recommended daily allowance and then splashed its boxes with a yellow banner: "Now HELPS SUPPORT YOUR CHILD'S IMMUNITY." Nutrition experts such as Marion Nestle begged to differ: "All nutrients are involved in immune function," wrote Nestle in her blog post on the topic. "But is it remotely possible that Cocoa Krispies might protect your child against colds or swine flu? I wish."

Says Jack Gwaltney Jr., "If things like dietary supplements and cereals contained some kind of magic that made you develop antibodies instantly [targeted at the particular virus in question], that would be wonderful. But that's not the case." Most of the products on the market make the simple blanket claim of goosing immunity. Even if they contain ingredients that have been shown to alter components of the immune system, there's no evidence that they actually bolster protection against infection. Which cells are best to boost and to what number? No one really knows. We do know that boosting any old element in the immune system is not necessarily a good thing. If the miserable symptoms of a cold are actually the result of your body's own inflammatory responses, the notion of enhancing these responses to prevent or shorten colds doesn't make scientific sense. In fact, given what we know about the genesis of cold symptoms, the last thing you may want to do is upset the balance in your body by boosting the number of proinflammatory cytokines. Birgit Winther once described to me what happened when a colleague of hers at the University of Copenhagen decided to try taking some immune-enhancing drugs to get over a cold. "He told me he had never been so sick in his whole life," Winther recalls. "This makes sense," she says. "If we get our white blood cells to work better, we're going to have a stronger immune response and more exaggerated symptoms."

So, what is normally the upshot of the body's natural response to a cold virus?

*   *   *

Sneezing, the "Trumpet of Nature." Most languages possess an onomatopoetic word for the proverbial sharp intake of air and its explosive release. In Hebrew it's *apchi*, in Swedish *atjo*, in Russian *apchkhi*, in Japanese *hakushon*, in Korean *achee*, in Cypriot Greek *apshoo*. Sneezing, the "trumpet of nature," or sternutation, as it's formally known, can be like scratching—one of nature's sweetest gratifications—unless it's relentless, as is often the case with hay fever or severe colds. It tends to peak on the second or third day of a cold.

As Sir Thomas Browne told us in the 17th century, "the custom of saluting or blessing upon that motion" has a long and illustrious history, in part arising from its status as an omen, good or bad, and also from its link with chest ailments "wherein Sternutation proved mortal, and such as Sneezed, died."

In days of yore, a good *ah-choo!* was seen as a necessary ejection of a noxious vapor from the brain. (You can see the point; sneezing can feel purging or exorcising.) But now we know that it has much more plebian origins, triggered by inflammatory chemicals in the nose. These spark sensory nerves that carry the sneeze message to a special center in the medulla area of the brain stem, where the sneeze reflex is controlled—and where older antihistamines such as Benadryl work to calm sneezing.

It's not easy to stimulate the sneeze reflex, says Gwaltney. He should know. He has tried everything from tickling people's noses to having them snort pepper. The only method that works consistently is putting histamine on the lining of the nose. So sneezing would appear to be triggered by histamine. "Yet there's no sign of a boost in histamine in nasal secretions during a cold as there is during allergic rhinitis," Gwaltney points out. "Instead, it may be that during a cold, the body becomes more sensitive to the histamine that's normally present in the nose."

Once stimulated, the sneeze center triggers a reflex activation of facial nerves and respiratory muscles in the diaphragm and the chest: the eyes close, the face grimaces, air is inspired and then quickly, explosively expired, and the nose runs freely.

Congestion and Runny Nose. The average cold sufferer easily uses some 20 or 30 tissues a day to mop up the cascade of free-flowing nasal fluids. Ancients believed this serum leaked into the nose from the cranial cavity, filtering through Swiss cheese–like holes in the skull's cribriform plate, just above the nose. In truth, the unlovely drip is made of watery fluid from mucous glands and from plasma that oozes through nasal blood capillary walls when inflammatory mediators make the cells in the capillary walls "unzip," opening at their junctions just enough to let out plasma but not red blood cells. The ooze, which increases a hundredfold during a cold, carries a complex mix of inflammatory chemicals that stimulate the pain nerve fibers in and around the nose and irritate the skin.

It's a surprise to learn that the glands in our nose and sinuses normally make as much as a couple of quarts of mucus a day—a viscous mix of water, lipids, carbohydrates, and glycoproteins called mucins—which keep our nasal membranes moist and sweep germs and dirt from airways into pharynx and down to stomach. (We typically swallow around a quart a day.) We're blissfully unaware of all this until the body boosts its output during a cold.

Though mucus is a magical and essential mix, I treasure it not—from my nose or any other. Apparently there are some who do. In the winter of 2008 Scarlett Johansson appeared on the *Tonight Show with Jay Leno* to promote her latest film despite suffering from a wicked cold she said she had caught from her costar. Never one to undervalue her own productions, she decided at the spur of the moment to auction off her used tissue on eBay. Bidding began at $0.99. Some 83 bids later, the item sold for $5,300. To charity went the proceeds from what must be far and away the world's most valuable snot rag.

Contrary to popular belief, drinking milk will not increase the volume of secretions during a cold, and color changes do not signify serious trouble. The green mucus that often graces children's noses (and when it appeared in my young girls, used to send my sister-in-law in search of surgical masks for her own family) is not a sign of bacterial infection, as some doctors think. Rather, it reflects the might of the immune response: as more and more of those white blood cells known as polys are recruited to the nose, the color of the mucus changes from clear to yellow to green. The cells carry green iron-containing enzymes, which give the fluid that olive hue.

If you're convinced that your child's cold-ridden nose is runnier than yours, you're right. Children have the same number of mucous glands as adults but a smaller mucosal area in the nose, and thus diminished capacity to transport the mucus toward the back of the throat; hence the copious stream. A drippy nose is no cause for worry in a child unless it's persistently runny on one side only. That would suggest that a pea or pencil eraser or other small object is lodged in that nostril; the secretions are the body's desperate efforts to eject it.

Why is a runny nose cause for such distress? As the writer Margaret Visser points out, "Ours is a culture that is unusually determined to distinguish between liquid and solid. We easily dislike anything that falls between the two categories, especially if the substance is bodily: tears, freely running, are fine; spit or snot, which we describe as runny, are not." Also, a runny nose calls undue attention to an appendage many of us would prefer to forget—bulbous and reddened in its harbor, snug in the center of the face. (If you're feeling this way, remember Gogol's tale of poor Kovalyov, who discovers one day that his nose has left him to pursue its own career, leaving its crestfallen former owner with a face flat and barren.)

Incidentally, the runny nose that plagues us when we walk or jog or ski in frigid weather is an altogether different beast from the runny nose of a cold. Cold-induced rhinitis, also known as skier's nose, can be triggered by exercise, stress, spicy food, and especially exposure to dry, chilly air. "It serves no particular purpose," says Steven Churchill, a biological anthropologist at Duke University, "but it is a byproduct of a critical function: warming and humidifying inspired air on its way to the lungs."

To digress for a moment: The air that reaches your lungs must be at body temperature and 100 percent absolute humidity. When inspired air is very cold, your nose has to work overtime to condition it. When you inhale, the cold, dry air comes in contact with moist tissue inside your nose. The blood vessels in your turbinates dilate, your mucosal tissue swells, and your glands secrete extra mucus; this moisture evaporates and humidifies the air before it goes to the lungs. As you exhale, the newly heated, moist air coming back out from the lungs cools again. The moisture recondenses onto the mucosa, where it's then in place for the next breath. The problem is that some noses are so good at the task that on a cold day, the moisture recapture mechanism operates faster than our ability to reincorporate the excess, so it accumulates on the inside of the nasal passage, and the embarrassing flow begins.

As Churchill has discovered, what makes one nose more likely to run than another has a lot to do with the airflow created by its inner features. This increases the exposure of moving air to the mucosa, facilitating the heat and moisture exchange.

It's worth lingering here for a moment, as Churchill's research is a good example of the lengths to which scientists will go to unpick the secrets of the nose. To fathom how the nose's architectural features influence airflow, Churchill devised a most unusual model. He procured ten cadavers—six males and four females—held their heads upside down, blocked their throats with clay, and poured molten metal inside their noses. He worked the metal around until the nasal passageway was full, then he cut that section out and macerated it to remove all the tissue. From this metal positive of the air space, he created an anatomically accurate acrylic model of the nasal passageway. Finally, he suspended the model in anatomical position in a tank of water and then suctioned dye-tinted water through the nose while video-recording the flow.

In this way, Churchill discovered that the turbulent flow that enhances moisture exchange was most pronounced in noses with larger passageways and downwardly directed nares. This fits with what scientists know about the geographic variation in nasal form as an adaptation to climate. "Populations adapted to cold or dry environments tend to have larger, more protrusive noses with downward nares," says Churchill; "those adapted to hot, humid environments have smaller, flatter noses and more anteriorly directed nares." So, should you find yourself in sudden need to put nose to sleeve despite being cold-free and in good health, by all means, blame your forebears.

As for the effect of nose size and shape on colds: Ron Eccles recently reviewed their possible influence on susceptibility to colds and other respiratory diseases and found no link. "Nasal proportions are important aesthetically," he concluded, "but appear to have little relevance to the rhinologist."

A typical cold victim blows her nose an average of 45 times

during the first three days of illness, especially after sneezing. As we've learned, hard blowing is not a good idea. It won't alleviate the stuffy, blocked feeling that stifles breathing, as this is not the product of excess mucus but a result of those swelling blood vessels in the spongy turbinates of the nose. Perhaps more important, studies show that forceful nose blowing propels viscous nasal fluid, with its load of viruses, bacteria, and inflammatory chemicals, into the sinuses, where secondary bacterial infections may take hold. It's best to be gentle with nose blowing and to blow one nostril at a time.

In truth, colds almost inevitably involve the sinuses, but only rarely (in about 2 percent of cases) do they lead to secondary infections. Some time ago, Jack Gwaltney Jr. used computed tomography scans to peer into the sinus cavities of people with early colds. He discovered to his surprise that 87 percent of people with recent colds had abnormalities in their sinuses—thick material adhering to the walls and blocked drainage passages. (These passages are normally the diameter of pencil lead, so it doesn't take much to obstruct them. Mucus normally moves through them at the blinding rate of a centimeter a minute.) The vast majority of these abnormalities completely resolved or improved markedly within a couple of weeks, without antibiotic treatment. This is not to say that people don't develop bacterial sinusitis as a complication of colds, "just that sinus involvement is part and parcel of a normal cold, almost an integral part of the disease," says Gwaltney.

Sinus pain may arise from pressure changes in the air chambers or in the blood vessels draining the sinuses, which are laced with sensory nerves.

All of this clogging and congestion makes some people lose their sense of smell. The comedian Henny Youngman supposedly endured such deprivation when the first Smell-O-Vision film was released in 1960. The film boasted a smell track that activated vials of scents like garlic, pipe tobacco, and boot polish. But Youngman gave it this review: "I didn't understand the picture. I had a cold."

Cough. Who hasn't been in the agonizing position—in a concert hall, at a meeting, seated at a formal dining table—of trying to stifle a cough? It has the same effect as holding down the lid of an overboiling pot. There's no denying the physics of it. Coughing is an irrepressible response to irritation in the sensory receptors of the throat, below the larynx. It's a protective reaction, designed to blow the irritant, whether meat or mucus, up and out of the airway. But it's no simple reflex. The stimulated nerves send a message to the cough center in the brain stem. There's a sudden inspiration of air, followed by a quick squeeze of muscle in the diaphragm. The glottis, the opening of the larynx, closes briefly to boost air pressure. As the glottis suddenly reopens, a turbulent blast of air is released from the lungs at speeds of more than 2,500 centimeters per second, tearing off excessive secretions and anything else that needs to be expelled.

However, cold-induced coughs, which occur in about a third of cold sufferers, are often dry and unproductive, serving no useful purpose and disrupting everything from sleep to that exquisite Bach cantata. They're caused by the body's inflammatory response spreading to the larynx. Those pesky inflammatory mediators may "tickle" the sensory nerve endings in our airways, making them hyper-reactive, so they respond to stimuli they would normally ignore—like simple saliva. Cough frequency tends to peak between noon and 6 p.m. and to ebb between midnight and 6 a.m. The severity of a cough generally crests around day four of a cold, though one study showed that in some 25 percent of people, it will hang on for up to two weeks. As Ogden Nash put it, "Just when you think you're through coughing, there's another cough in the offing."

The most irritating thing is the inability to control the impulse—a phenomenon that has driven some concert- and theater-goers to carry an ample supply of lozenges to pass out to offending audience members. The *New Yorker*'s "Talk of the Town" once told a tale of such a Vicks vigilante, an elderly lady who for two decades occupied the same balcony seat for Friday afternoon concerts at Carnegie Hall. At one Friday concert, when a woman nearby was seized with a fit of coughing, the lady reached into her bag and passed a tablet down the aisle. The woman gratefully swallowed it and ceased her disruptive hacking. After the concert, the elderly lady discovered that she had accidentally given the woman a florist's tablet for prolonging the life of cut flowers.

Some blame a persistent cough on postnasal drip, that film of mucus traveling steadily down the back of the throat at the rate of a quart a day, which may produce what is best described by a 19th-century otolaryngologist as that "sense of fullness deeply seated in the back of the nose, with constant stinging and tickling sensation about the uvula [and]...palate." We all have postnasal mucus and normally swallow it without knowing it; during a cold, it may accumulate, causing irritation and cough. But others do not hold with the postnasal notion. Phil Jones of the University Hospital of South Manchester, for example, writes, "The chest physicians—bless their little cotton socks—still seem to believe in excess mucus collecting on the uvula, biding its time until the vocal folds gape beneath and then (holding its nose no doubt) jumping off and diving into the larynx." Postnasal drip can be linked with cough without being the cause of it, says Jones. When it comes to a cold, those inflammatory chemicals may just linger for unknown reasons, inflaming airways and obliterating arias.

*   *   *

Stopped-up Ears. In some 75 percent of rhinovirus infections, people develop abnormal middle ear pressure around the second day of their colds—not generally a major concern unless you're an airman or an astronaut. During World War II, James Lovelock was asked to try to prevent the spread of colds among American crewmen flying B-17s over German-occupied Europe. One may wonder why anything as trivial as a cold was worth wasting time on during war, he writes in his memoirs. In fact it was no bureaucratic blunder but an effort to address the excruciating ear pain caused by the common cold for crew members flying in an unpressurized airplane at 20,000 feet. The ear pain resulted from the distension of the eardrum when the congestion from a cold prevented the normal release of excess pressure in the middle ear as the plane ascended.

The pressure problem arises when swelling or congestion blocks the eustachian tubes. These are the narrow passageways that connect the hollow chamber of the middle ear with the back of the nose. The tube is closed until swallowing pulls it open and allows fresh air into the chamber, which equalizes your middle ear pressure with the air pressure outside your head. But if the tube becomes blocked, the air pressure doesn't equalize properly. Normally the abnormal pressure resolves on its own as congestion subsides. But if the blockage is prolonged, fluid drawn into the chamber can cause infection.

Most of us have experienced ear discomfort while flying with a cold, though nothing like that suffered by those B-17 crewmen, thanks to the equalized air pressure in modern aircraft cabins, which rarely falls below the pressure experienced at 5,000 feet. Still, flying with a roaring cold is no fun. The pressure changes with ascent and descent can cause serious sinus headaches or trap gas in the middle ear space, creating ear pain or dizziness. It may help to take an oral decongestant or nasal decongestant spray 30 minutes before takeoff, which can help shrink your nasal mucosa enough to let air into your sinuses and allow them to drain. If you're not too stuffed up, you can equalize the pressure by swallowing frequently, chewing gum, or performing a gentle Valsalva maneuver, holding your nose and mouth closed while attempting to exhale every 30 seconds or so, generating pressure against your mouth and glottis until your ears pop. To ease ear pain for babies and toddlers during descent, it's helpful to have the babies nurse or suck a pacifier or bottle while upright to help open the eustachian tubes. Older children can drink from a cup.

The Axis of Evil: Headache, Malaise, and Poor Performance. "If you told me the world will be at an end to-morrow, I should just say, 'Will it?' I have not volition enough left to dot my *i*'s,...my brains are gone out to see a poor relation in Moorfields, and they did not say when they'd come back again; my skull is a Grub Street attic to let."

Charles Lamb's description may be a little overblown, but we all know that unpleasant feeling of lassitude that often accompanies a cold—the mild headache, fatigue, and loss of appetite. About half of people with colds get a headache early in their infection, probably as a result of those troublesome proinflammatory cytokines acting in the brain. In children, they can cause fever.

Fortunately, symptoms of headache and achiness decline rapidly after a day or two, whereas the malaise—the irritability, loss of interest in pleasurable activities such as eating and socializing, inability to concentrate, disturbed sleep, in short the "blahs"—can last much longer, wreaking havoc with our good humor.

Frank Sinatra with a cold was "Picasso without paint, Ferrari without fuel—only worse," wrote Gay Talese in his famous profile of the legendary singer. Not only did a cold render Sinatra's voice weak and uncertain but it so utterly fouled his mood that it caused "a kind of psychosomatic nasal drip within dozens of people who work for him."

Even for those of us who don't croon for a living, sneezing and wheezing with cold can sabotage performance and mess with mood. Research shows that when we have colds, we feel dopier and less alert, with more "negative" attitudes about the world. In 2007, Denise Janicki-Deverts and her colleagues exposed a large group of healthy adult volunteers to an experimental rhinovirus strain; then, during an ensuing six-day period of quarantine, measured their daily production of cold-induced proinflammatory cytokines. They also measured the volunteers' daily mood states with the help of both a "positive scale" (assessing vigor, calmness, and well-being: How full of pep are you? How much at ease? How cheerful or happy?) and a "negative scale" (assessing depression, anxiety, and anger: How sad are you? How tense? How hostile?) The team found that higher production of three cytokines on one day was linked to lower scores on the positive scale the following day (though not higher scores on the negative scale).

Colds equal less pep and good cheer. Big surprise.

As for physical feats, colds don't seem to hamper lung function or capacity for exercise, but runners beware: some studies suggest that they can alter so-called kinematics—stride length and frequency—raising the risk of injury. Nonetheless most doctors encourage exercise during a cold, as it tends to make us feel better—perhaps because it dilates blood vessels and increases blood flow.

Mental performance is another matter. Colds hinder our ability to carry out certain tasks, especially simple psychomotor tasks that require the coordination of sensory and motor skills. Having a cold slows reaction times and disrupts hand-eye coordination, so we do worse at jobs that require tracking a moving target or manual dexterity (for instance, moving pegs quickly from one set of holes to another). One study found that colds slow our response to unexpected events and interfere with our ability to sustain attention. The take-home message of this research? If you're suffering sniffles, it's a good idea to resist your urge not only for archery and pegboards but also for driving.

As for how we do at higher mental functions such as reasoning, learning, and memory when we're under the weather, the news is mixed. Colds don't seem to impinge on our ability to reason or to recall lists of words or strings of digits. But studies suggest they can interfere with learning and recall of more complex material, such as stories. When people have a story read to them and then are asked to recall information from it, those down with colds tend to remember random details, while healthy people recall what's most germane. This suggests that colds may affect our ability to analyze and process relevant information. They also appear to slow our mental processing during cognitive tasks. In a 2007 study, Romola Bucks of the University of Western Australia and her colleagues found that colds reduce the speed with which we remember things. Though our accuracy doesn't suffer much, we're slower to recognize and remember both words and pictures. Perhaps not surprisingly, the effect is more pronounced in older participants. "What all of this tells us is that even very mild infections can affect our mental skills," says Bucks. "The slowing effect might be an adaptive response: That is, we slow up in order to maintain accuracy." So when you have a cold, you should be gentle on yourself, she advises, and realize that mental tasks, whether they involve memory or emotions, may take longer and feel harder.

Just why a cold in the nose influences the workings of the

brain is still a mystery. The simple distraction of annoying symptoms may be the culprit. Or perhaps it's those mischievous cytokines. "It appears likely that cytokines directly or indirectly are related to some of the 'head'/'brain' symptoms of a common cold," says Bernhard Baune, a professor of psychiatry at James Cook University in Australia. The particulars are not well understood, but some cytokines present during colds may affect learning and memory consolidation—the changes in the brain that allow memories to be more permanently stored. Or it could be that the link is something as simple as lost sleep.

One study led by Christopher Drake, an investigator at the Henry Ford Hospital Sleep Disorders Center, showed that people suffering cold symptoms sleep an average of 23 minutes less per night than healthy people and, perhaps more important, get 36 minutes less consolidated sleep. In people with colds, "sleep is fragmented, with frequent shifts to lighter stages of sleep," says Drake. The 20 or 30 minutes of lost sleep may not seem like much, but Drake believes it could affect brain function, especially if a cold is lengthy and sleep debt accumulates. To help minimize any sleep-disturbance effects and ensure adequate overall sleep time, Drake suggests spending time in bed during a cold.

To what end is all of this misery and poor showing? What a waste if our inflammatory engines revving in high gear were all for naught. The fact is, certain cold symptoms may do some good, and some experts suggest that squelching them altogether—if such a thing were possible—may not be such a good idea.

Malaise, for instance, serves a purpose by telling the body to rest and preserve its resources. The lethargy and social withdrawal, known as "sick behavior," is meant to force us to reorganize our priorities to promote recovery. A little depressed activity is a survival mechanism, says Andrew Miller, a professor of psychiatry at the Emory University School of Medicine; it's common in the animal kingdom. The squirrel goes unchased, the nut unburied, the date book unopened so that the body can conserve energy to heal itself.

As for sneezing, coughing, and runny nose, "they are all part of the body's effort to get rid of the virus, to wash it out," says Birgit Winther. The inflammatory response that underlies these symptoms results in the body's production of such antiviral substances as interferon, which fights the virus immediately, and eventually produces antibodies, which appear about two weeks after infection and protect against reinfection. "The mechanical methods work first; then the body's own antivirals and antibodies," explains Winther. "It's best not to take away the inflammatory response completely, or you could block this antiviral and antibody response, too," she says, "actually boosting viral replication and, perhaps, prolonging symptoms."

This is all well and good except for a few small hitches, says Jack Gwaltney Jr. "Runny nose is good for ridding the nose of things like ragweed pollen and bacteria," he explains. "These are responses the body developed a long time ago, before respiratory viruses came along. They don't work well for ridding the body of viruses, which are cloistered in the cells of the nose, which you don't particularly want to get rid of."

Then there's the issue of that 25 percent of people who seem to get cold infections but not suffer symptoms. These people seem to be able to rid themselves of cold infections—and eventually to produce antibodies to the virus in question—without ever suffering the normal, annoying symptoms of a cold.

Some years ago Gwaltney conducted a small, informal study to explore a deep hunch about this. He invited several people who claimed never to catch colds to participate in the 15-year study, among them his late first wife. ("She just didn't get colds," he told me. "It was pretty irritating.") Gwaltney drew blood from his volunteers to determine that none of the subjects had been exposed to 10 or 12 strains of rhinovirus as measured by the presence of antibodies. Then, over the 15-year period, he kept records of the occurrence of colds in these subjects. At the end of the period, he once again measured for the presence of antibodies to the different rhinovirus strains. It turned out that the subjects who never got colds had the same prevalence of antibodies as those who did get colds. In other words, these non-cold-suffering subjects had become infected and made antibodies, but not one of them suffered symptoms. "They were infected all right," says Gwaltney, but their infections were "silent"—present but completely symptomless.

This explains in part why cold viruses seem less transmissible than they really are. The bugs can spread fairly easily, but their contagion does not always lead to colds themselves. And here's a paradox: "It may be that these symptomless people are not making the normal amounts of inflammatory mediators that cause cold symptoms," says Gwaltney. "If that's the case, then there may be a real irony here: people with more active immune systems may be more prone to having cold symptoms than people with less active immune systems." Which rather turns on its head the myth that susceptibility to colds arises from a weakened immune system.

The experience of a cold, it seems, may be determined not so much by the nature of the virus but by the nature of you. As Louis Pasteur once said, "The germ is nothing; the terrain is everything."

Chapter 5

THE TERRAIN

Has a woman who knew that she was well dressed ever caught a cold?

FRIEDRICH NIETZSCHE

We all know people, well dressed or not, who almost never get colds; and on the flip side, people who seem to succumb to every bug that comes down the runway. Maybe your spouse is of the resilient sort, and you, cold-prone. When it comes to resisting bugs, did you just draw a short genetic straw? Is your "enhanced" vulnerability inevitable, or are there things you can do to reduce it?

The good news is that in almost everyone, susceptibility to colds declines over time. People over age 50, for instance, catch colds only half as often as teenagers. The advantage of the older crowd is partly due to a lifetime of exposure to colds and the resulting gift of antibodies to many common cold viruses. But it's also about human nature.

Children are walking cold magnets. Newborns may get a dose of temporary immunity from their moms. Mother's milk definitely helps stave off infections in babies. Breast milk carries not only antibodies developed by the mother in response to her own colds but also a miraculous mixture of carbohydrates, proteins, and other elements, which are passed on to the nursing baby and protect its airways. In the first four months of life, respiratory bugs of all types are less common in breast-fed than formula-fed babies, including that scourge, ear infections. But by the time infants are six months old, they're susceptible to all variety of bugs, and by one year of age, a new phenomenon kicks in: world exploration and the exposure it brings. To investigate their environment, children employ their most useful tools: fingers, eyes, mouth, and even nose. Studies show that for one-year-olds, the average number of hand-to-mouth and object-to-mouth (and often, to nose) episodes per hour is around 64. By age four, this drops to around 10. But still.

Then around comes day care or preschool, those "hot zones," as Harley Rotbart calls them, "where kids and germs gather in high numbers." Rotbart speaks often to parent groups, and among the most common question he receives is this: Are my kids getting sicker in day care than if I kept them at home? The answer is yes. But there's a silver lining, says Rotbart. "They'll have plenty of natural immunity by the time they go to school. Kids who are kept at home for their early years won't have as much of this immunity because they've had fewer exposures and will get these bugs when they start kindergarten. By the time kids are ten years old, they all end up with the same repertoire of exposure regardless of how they spent their first five years."

Another common query: Does it help to bundle them up in cold weather? We know that cold doesn't cause colds (viruses do). But does being chilly make one more susceptible? Though most research dismisses the old folklore about catching a cold from catching a chill, a study or two still lingers attempting to link the two. At least one new theory suggests that the cooling of the nose that takes place in winter lowers resistance to infection by viruses already present in the nose, allowing them to replicate. A related experiment at the Common Cold Centre in Cardiff, United Kingdom, in 2005 looked at the effects of foot chilling in a study of 180 students. The researchers asked 90 volunteers to sit with their bare feet in a bucket of ice water for 20 minutes while another 90 students sat in their socks and shoes with the feet in an empty bucket. No one in either group caught cold instantly. Over the next five days, however, more than three times as many students from the chilled group reported cold symptoms compared with the nonchilled group. The researchers proposed that chilling the feet causes the blood vessels in the nose to constrict, inhibiting the immune response to viruses already present in the nose. But as critics are quick to point out, the trial has serious limitations. There were no virology studies—the researchers made no effort to determine whether any of the subjects actually had infections or were just experiencing symptoms. Moreover, the study wasn't blinded (the chilly- and toasty-footed knew who they were), so the self-reported results were potentially biased.

Like most experts, Ron Turner of the University of Virginia is not convinced that there's anything to the old wives' tale. "Exposure to cold has nothing to do with catching a cold," he says. Colds are more common in fall and winter because the cooler, wetter weather drives people indoors, where viruses may more easily jump from one person to the next. Relative humidity may also play into the picture. Rhinoviruses prefer a relatively low level of humidity, around 20 to 40 percent, which is more common in the colder months. But the very real peak in colds in September and early January is likely due to the return of students to schools and colleges after the summer and winter break. Densely packed day-care centers, schools, and colleges provide an ideal breeding ground for bugs, which then radiate out into the community.

Age aside, why susceptibility to the common cold varies so much among the general population has been a stubbornly persistent riddle. In the first part of the 20th century, a debate raged over whether there was such a thing as a "cold constitution"—the opposite, presumably, of what my mother used to call an iron constitution. In the 1930s, scientists probed possible links between physical or ethnic characteristics and resilience to colds. One group went so far as to look for ties between susceptibility and eye color or ethnic heritage. Not surprisingly, they found no differences in incidence, severity, or character of colds between Jews and non-Jews or between blue-eyed and brown-eyed people.

A decade later, a Boston team took another tack: if there was in fact a cold constitution, they reasoned, then the number of colds a person gets from year to year should hold fairly constant. Indeed, when the team analyzed a group of boys at Phillips Exeter Academy, they found that each boy tended to have the same number of colds year after year, and the numbers varied considerably from boy to boy. But was the difference a matter of constitution or environment? Because the setting for the study, the academy, was a constant for all the boys, the group favored a constitutional factor "not as yet defined." This was before the discovery of DNA, genes, and the whirligig of inflammatory cells and molecules involved in the body's response to a cold. But the researchers were right. In later years, environmental factors such as cold, dampness, and air pollution would be largely ruled out as players.

The results of the Exeter inquiry tracked nicely with a big epidemiological study conducted in the late 1960s, the Seattle

Virus Watch, which looked at patterns of infection within 65 families. The Virus Watch tested the families for cold-virus infection and recorded the presence of illness. It turned out that some families had symptoms with every infection, whereas other families, though infected, never suffered any symptoms at all. Five families were plagued by 38 infections over the four-year course of the study; all 38 resulted in illness. In three other families, 20 infections were recorded, but none resulted in illness.

Not long ago, Thomas Ball decided to reexamine the constitutional question in light of new science. "I became darned intrigued by the common cold and the idea that there might be constitutional factors that made some kids more susceptible to it," says Ball, now a professor of pediatrics at the University of Arizona. "I come from healthy stock myself; in 22 years as a pediatrician, I've hardly gotten sick at all."

Ball and his colleagues looked at a population of more than 1,000 children in day-care centers and schools in Tucson over time to see whether the likelihood of developing frequent common colds persisted throughout childhood and whether there might be any chemical markers for greater susceptibility. In 2002, Ball reported his finding that, indeed, children who got lots of colds when they were toddlers were twice as likely to get lots of colds through their school years compared with schoolchildren who had only occasional colds when they were little.

"And when we took a peek at the only chemical marker we had at the time, interferon, lo and behold, we found there was something immunologically different about these kids," says Ball. The children who had greater susceptibility had blood cells that responded to stimuli (such as the cold virus) with lower levels of the antiviral chemical. "This was a pretty crude marker," he admits. "We have better ones now. But it was an indicator that some kind of host factor difference was at work.

"If you had asked me 15 years ago, I would have told you quite simply that viruses cause the cold, and that it's just the luck of nature whether you get a bad one or a milder case or no cold at all," says Ball. "Now I think host factors are very significant, maybe 40 to 60 percent of the equation. It's clear to me that there really are clusters of kids who are more susceptible—Velcro kids, who catch everything."

In the past 5 or 10 years, we've discovered genetic variations that may account for these disparities in our susceptibility—differences in the little cell receptors to which rhinoviruses attach, for instance, and in the nature and amounts of inflammatory chemicals we make. Genetic differences in the cell receptor may affect your likelihood of getting infected to begin with; differences in the expression of cytokines, those natural body chemicals that cause cold symptoms, may determine whether you suffer congestion and other cold ills. Learning this has been a slow process—one gene at a time.

Ron Turner has a dream to speed things up. "Up until now," he says, "we've only looked at individual genes. We've said, okay, interleukin 8 is an important cytokine, so we'll look at differences in that gene." Turner would like to search the whole genome in one fell swoop for all of the genetic variations associated with cold infection and illness. "We would have to look at lots of people and compare their genetic blueprint in lots of different places all at once," he says. "A genome-wide scan would be expensive, but we have the ability to do it. It would involve collecting DNA from a large group of volunteers, 800 or so, and infecting them with virus. Most would get infected, and some would get sick (around 70 percent). There would also be variation in the severity of illness. By scanning and comparing whole genomes, we could look for differences and mismatches in SNPs [single-nucleotide polymorphisms, or little variations in DNA] consistent with the findings of differences in people's infection and illness."

A big, ambitious study such as this could answer big questions about susceptibility: What genes are different in the people who don't get infected? And in those who get infected but don't get ill? And how about those who suffer especially severe symptoms or go on to get complications from colds, such as sinus or ear infections? "We could find all of the SNPs that predict who's going to get infected and who's going to get ill," says Turner. "There could be a hundred things involved, everything from the inflammatory response to factors that seem utterly unrelated."

It's the unexpected players in disease that are often the most helpful in developing treatments. Not long ago, scientists conducted this sort of broad comparative genome study for macular degeneration, a progressive eye disease. They found a surprise. "When they looked at the whole genomes of those with the disease and those without," says Turner, "what fell out as the difference was the gene for complement, an immune protein. Who knew?" Suddenly, there was another potential strategy for slowing the disease—developing agents that inhibit or block complement.

This kind of study of the genetics of colds that could yield such helpful targets is probably not far off. But as Turner points out, what happens in the human body is never strictly a function of genes alone. There's all that other stuff that's going on, both within the body and outside it.

Fatigue, for instance. Ask around, and many people will tell you that they get a cold when they're run-down or have had a bad night's sleep. According to Jack Gwaltney Jr., just feeling tired has little impact on susceptibility. Over a 10-year period, Gwaltney infected more than 300 student volunteers and found that fatigue had no effect on whether they came down with a cold.

Sleep deprivation is another issue. Anecdotes abound of pulling an all-nighter as a student, or as a parent, being cheated of sleep by small children, and 36 hours later, coming down with a cold. New research suggests a sound link between sleep and susceptibility. In 2009, Sheldon Cohen and his team at Carnegie Mellon University found that people who slept fewer than seven hours a night were three times more likely to develop a cold than those who slept eight hours or more. Sleep efficiency, the percentage of time in bed actually spent asleep, had an even bigger impact. "Even small losses from minor disruptions—trouble dozing off or waking up through the night—had an effect," he says; people who lost just 2 to 8 percent of their total sleep time (that's about 10 to 40 minutes for the average 8-hour night) had up to five times the risk of getting sick compared with those who fell asleep quickly and slept soundly. Just what could explain this link between sleep and colds is still a mystery. Cohen speculates that it may involve those proinflammatory chemicals that cause cold symptoms. Previous research has shown that sleep deprivation enhances proinflammatory processes in the body. It may be that when we don't get sufficient sleep, we don't properly regulate our immune systems.

Stress is likely another factor in susceptibility. Most of us are only too aware that when we're "stressed out," we seem especially vulnerable to bugs. But what exactly does it mean to be stressed out? The expression is so overused, it has worn thin. People talk about stress as if it were a single, monolithic entity. It's not. There's tremendous individual variation in the way people cope with stressors. For some, even the mildest hassle causes deep anxiety and stress. Others are utterly unfazed even by severe stressors that would send most of us over the edge. Moreover, there are certain kinds of stress that are actually good for the body. Acute stress, the short-term variety that comes with confronting your boss, say, or giving a lecture, can do wonders for the body. It elicits the stress response, known as the fight-or-flight reaction, which sharpens your senses and steps up your heart rate and blood pressure in preparation for short-term challenges. While the stress response may guzzle energy, it can also boost performance and enhance your sense of physical and mental well-being. But only if it's put into play for brief periods.

What makes us feel stressed out is chronic stress, the mounting pressure we feel from exposure to long-term stressors such as perpetual worry about work, debt, marital issues, or illness in the family. This kind of chronic stress mounts, causing us to lose sleep, stop exercising, and eat poorly—all of which puts us at higher risk of illness. It's doubtful that brief bouts of stress, such as putting in overtime at your job for a week or two or having dinner with your in-laws, is going to make you more susceptible to infection. But longer-lasting stress—living in a war zone or in extreme poverty, for instance, or the death of a close relative or chronic illness in a spouse or child—may indeed be a threat to your health.

People have embraced the link between even mild stress and susceptibility to colds at least since the 1950 debut of *Guys and Dolls*, in which Adelaide laments, "Just from waiting around for that little band of gold, a girl can develop a cold." But because stress is so individual and variable, the link with illness was viewed as soft science—intuitive and anecdotal but hard to prove.

That is, until Sheldon Cohen tackled the problem. In the early 1980s, Cohen was a young psychologist interested in a theory that chronic noise in city environments might impair reading ability in children. When he tested his theory, he found that not only did relentless noise interfere with the children's learning of speech sounds, it also raised their blood pressure. How could a stressor such as noise "get inside the body," as Cohen expressed it? Could stressors have other health effects? Could they compromise the body's ability to fight infection?

A golden opportunity to sort out these questions presented itself when Cohen was introduced to David Tyrrell of the Common Cold Unit. "That was in the late 1980s," Cohen recalls. "At that time, it was hard to find scientists who were interested in the psychological aspects of illness. But Tyrrell was extremely supportive. He was not only a virologist but a physician. He had patients who said they thought their susceptibility to colds was related to stress. So he was open to this sort of study."

Tyrrell was indeed intrigued by the concept. "The whole idea that the mind could change virus infections, or be changed by them, seemed of crucial importance because it could be applied in so many other aspects of medicine," he wrote. He was happy to piggyback Cohen's psychological research on several studies at the CCU over a period of four years.

"It was really an accident that I ended up focusing on the cold," says Cohen. "But it was a good accident: the cold is a great experimental model because you can safely give the illness to people under controlled conditions. The CCU was an appealing place to work," he recalls, "very old-school British, with tea every afternoon." Between crumpets and scones, Cohen managed to produce what is considered the landmark study on stress and colds. He gave more than 300 healthy volunteers at the CCU a questionnaire about stressful events in their lives and then dosed them with cold viruses and watched to see who would get infected and who would show symptoms. The ones who fell sick were those who had scored high on his stress index. (This was true even when

Cohen factored in stress-related behaviors such as smoking, drinking, not exercising, and eating or sleeping poorly, all of which may affect susceptibility.) Some 47 percent of people in the highly stressed group got colds, compared with 27 percent in the least-stressed group. And the more stress a person was under, the worse the symptoms, as scientifically quantified by the amount of mucus he or she produced (extracted from those weighed tissues).

Over the past decade or so, Cohen has deliberately infected more than 1,000 healthy volunteers with cold virus to probe how psychological factors affect susceptibility and has published dozens of studies on the topic, many of them with Ron Turner and his group at UVA. When it comes to higher risk for colds, he has learned, the worst kind of stress you can have is the chronic kind—being out of a job or having lingering marriage trouble or difficulties with family or friends, particularly if they last for a month or longer. People enduring these kinds of chronic stressors are two to three times more likely to develop colds than those without them. The longer the stressful life event lasts, says Cohen, the greater your risk for developing a clinical illness.

Cohen has also turned up a strong correlation between socioeconomic status in childhood and susceptibility to colds. "It turns out that the number of years that your parents owned their own home during your childhood, before the age of 18, is negatively associated with whether you will develop a cold when exposed to a virus as an adult," he says—that is, the more years your parents were homeowners, the lower your risk of getting a lot of colds. "The most critical years are ages 0 to 6," he says. "If your parents did not own their home during these early years, you're at high risk—even if they did own their own home during your adolescent years. In other words, late ownership doesn't undo the damage. All of this is true no matter what your current adult socioeconomic status may be. So you have to hope you had rich parents!"

Cohen has also discovered that your perception of your own current socioeconomic status—rather than objective measures—to an extent predicts whether you'll develop a cold when exposed to a cold virus. In a 2008 study, Cohen used a new instrument to tap people's perceptions of how they rank in socioeconomic status in relation to others in their country. The tool is a simple picture of a ladder with 9 or 10 rungs. You're asked to place yourself on the ladder with respect to what you perceive as your standing in terms of income, education, and occupation. The lower you place yourself on that ladder, according to Cohen, the greater your risk of developing a cold when exposed to a cold virus—regardless of where you fall in objective terms. He suspects that the link here is poor sleep. "It could be that those low in subjective status worry more or feel a need to be more vigilant, which then influences their ability to sleep and, consequently, their susceptibility to disease."

Cohen has even unearthed support for the biblical proverb "A cheerful heart is good medicine." With the same experimental model he used for his stress studies, he looked at how our sociability and emotional style affect our risk of getting a cold. "The strongest, most consistent association is extraversion," he says. "Extraverts, people who seek out other people, are less susceptible to colds than introverts." The same is true for people with so-called positive emotional style (PES)—defined as having stable feelings of enthusiasm, high self-esteem, optimism, happiness, and mastery of their own lives. People with PES are less likely to catch colds. "The associations are really strong," says Cohen. "No matter the size of the study, these two factors are consistently and predictably linked to differences in cold susceptibility."

All of this raises a pretty basic question: What could be the biological mechanism underlying these links between stress, personality traits, and susceptibility? That is, how can external factors such as stressful life events or social connections get under the skin? Though the answer is still mysterious, clues are emerging.

We've all heard how stress suppresses immunity. There's good scientific evidence for this. The middleman is the stress hormone cortisol. People under stress make more cortisol as part of the fight-or-flight response. The cortisol boosts heart rate and blood pressure, preparing us to put up our dukes or run from danger. It also suppresses immunity. But there's a conundrum here. If inflammation and an overactive immune response drive cold symptoms, how can stress—which suppresses immunity—be at fault?

It turns out that one job of cortisol is to turn off the production of proinflammatory cytokines. If there's too much cortisol racing through the body, the hormone can't properly accomplish that task. So in effect, stress may not affect susceptibility to colds by suppressing the immune response. Quite the opposite, as Cohen explains. "Stress may short-circuit the body's ability to turn *off* production of proinflammatory cytokines, triggering a more severe symptomatic response." Indeed, Cohen's studies show that people under stress make more of the proinflammatory cytokine IL6. "So stressed people are not doing as good a job at regulating the release of inflammatory chemicals," he says. "They're releasing too much."

More proinflammatory cytokines, more cold symptoms. The same mechanism is at play in positive emotional style. Cohen has found that people with a positive emotional style produce fewer of the chemicals in response to cold viruses.

"When I first participated in these psychological studies, I was a little uncomfortable with the concept," recalls

Ron Turner. "It seemed a bit like pulling a rabbit from a hat. But now I believe there's really something to it. Just what, we still have to sort out. There may be subtle psychological factors involved. And the question inevitably arises: Is any of this modifiable? For instance, if you don't have the positive emotional style that makes you less susceptible to colds, can you change that?"

When I asked Cohen about this, he admitted that there was little data suggesting that people can modify these fundamental personality traits. "This is a very hot area in health psychology right now," he says. "There are some promising interventions with good short-term effects, and even some that last a long time. These mostly involve training people to think positively—writing positive, hopeful thoughts for 10 minutes a day, that sort of thing. But as yet, there's no really good evidence that people can change."

"I wouldn't be surprised if this sort of personality trait came down to a gene," says Turner. "You do see whole families where the trait seems to travel. So, people with a negative emotional style are stuck: 'Not only do I get depressed, but I get sick more easily. Now I'm really depressed!'"

Cohen is a little more optimistic. "We don't have a lot of evidence that health behaviors affect our susceptibility, but I wouldn't rule them out." People may not be able to flip their emotional style or personality type, but they can make some behavioral changes to reduce their susceptibility. For instance:

Catch Adequate Zzzs. When Cohen turned his spotlight on sleep in 2009, he found that people who slept for less than seven hours a night were three times more likely to get colds than longer sleepers. And those who didn't sleep well (spending less than 92 percent of their time actually asleep) were more than five times as likely to get a cold. Cohen speculates that sleep disturbance may influence the regulation of proinflammatory cytokines and other symptom mediators.

Snuff Out the Cigarettes. In the early 1990s, Cohen and his colleagues at the CCU probed the relationship between smoking and the incidence of colds. Smoking not only increased the risk of getting a cold (probably because it damages the delicate epithelial lining that defends our airways) but it worsened cold symptoms.

Exercise (But Not Too Much). Yet another reason to lace up the sneakers. People who exercise regularly—who get some kind of aerobic activity for 30 to 60 minutes a day, such as walking or running—report fewer colds than their sedentary peers and suffer fewer days of sickness from colds. A study by Charles Matthews, now of Vanderbilt University, showed that people who exercised for 30 minutes most days of the week averaged a little over one cold a year—a 23 percent lower rate than the average for the less-active group. The benefit was especially striking in the fall, when the more active group had a 30 percent reduction in risk of contracting a cold. While there were some limitations to the study (it relied on self-reports of colds collected every three months), the results are confirmed by earlier studies and by a more recent one that looked at the impact of moderate physical activity on the incidence of common colds among postmenopausal women. This study found that women who exercised regularly—for instance, walking briskly for 45 minutes a day—had about half the risk of colds compared to those who were not active. Moreover, the benefit appeared to increase over time and was strongest in the final quarter of the yearlong exercise program.

On the other hand, overdoing it—throwing yourself into

excessive, prolonged physical exertion (say, for longer than 90 minutes at a time)—may actually increase the risk of infection. Marathon runners who train more than 60 miles a week have twice the chance of coming down with a cold compared with those who train less than 20 miles a week. It may be that this sort of prolonged, heavy-duty exercise can affect the immune function of the respiratory tract, creating an "open window" through which viruses may gain a foothold.

Drink a Glass of Wine—Or Not. To Cohen's surprise, the two studies he conducted at the CCU showed that drinking moderately—one or two drinks day—actually diminished susceptibility. Nondrinkers were at greater risk of getting a cold. It's not clear why. "It could be that the types of people who drink are less susceptible for other reasons," Cohen suggests. Or there could be a direct link. Alcohol might somehow limit the replication of the viruses, or it might inhibit inflammatory processes. Either way, Cohen and his colleagues don't encourage drinking as a prophylactic or cure for the common cold, as the risks of consuming more than a drink or two a day far exceed the benefits in cold reduction.

Take a Vacation—Or Not. Vacation would seem to be good for the body, recharging the batteries and all that. For some, it does. But for others, holidays can be a source of considerable stress, with worries about travel, house and pet arrangements, etc., layered over the usual quotidian concerns. Even as simple a departure from routine as a weekend off can fray the nerves enough to boost susceptibility. For these folks, weekends can be stressful, and vacation, positively pathogenic, resulting in illness during precious time off. Ad Vingerhoets, a psychologist at Tilburg University in the Netherlands, calls this phenomenon "leisure sickness."

*   *   *

Expand Your Social Swath. People with diverse social networks—lots of different types of social relationships through marriage, work, and community, social, and religious groups—get fewer colds than those with small social circles. This is perhaps not so obvious: more contact with a broad range of people would seem to put you in the path of more cold viruses. But, says Cohen, it's the number of social roles that counts, not the number of individuals with whom you associate. In a 2004 study, Cohen found that people reporting only one to three types of relationships had more than four times the risk of frequent colds than people with six or more types of relationships. Not only were people with more types of social relationships less susceptible to developing colds, but they produced less mucus and shed less virus when they got them.

Don't Bother Trying to "Boost" Your Immunity with Vitamin, Herbs, or Other Supplements. Of course you want to eat well to keep your immune system healthy so that it properly regulates its responses. But there's little evidence that supplements do anything to prevent colds. (See chapter 6.) And given what we know about the genesis of cold symptoms, the last thing you may want to do is goose the number of immune cells in your body.

Chapter 6

KILLER COLDS

It's early spring 2007. At her boot camp at Lackland Air Force Base in Texas, 19-year-old airman Paige Villers is in her fifth week of basic training. This is "Warrior Week," a seven-day program that readies airmen for field conditions, complete with training in military survival skills, pitching tents, sleeping on cots, handling an M16 rifle, wading through waist-high water, getting by with too little sleep, and otherwise carrying out military duties in a stressful environment. Paige is an enthusiastic participant, a graduate of a high school in rural Norton, Ohio, who decided on the Air Force a day after graduating; she revels in the challenges and camaraderie of basic training. But during Warrior Week, she begins to feel sick, congested, and run-down.

It's not unusual for military recruits to suffer in this way. Some 9 out of 10 report cold symptoms at some point during their first months of basic training. Still, Villers is worried about passing the impending physical fitness test required for her to graduate that spring, so she consults the health clinic and is told she has allergies. She returns to training but begins to have difficulty breathing. When she takes her physical fitness test anyway, she fails the running section. A week later, she develops a high fever and checks into the Wilford Hall Medical Center with a diagnosis of mononucleosis. While at the hospital, she succumbs to a severe case of pneumonia that ravages her lungs. She is placed on a ventilator and enters a drug-induced coma. Her condition does not improve. Six weeks later, Paige Villers is dead. Probable diagnosis: viral pneumonia caused by a mutated version of a common cold virus known as adenovirus 14.

One of more than 50 strains of adenovirus, adenovirus 14 normally produces only a severe cold or sometimes conjunctivitis or gastroenteritis. But in 2006 and 2007, a new, more virulent variant of the virus emerged, causing serious respiratory illness in clusters of patients in Oregon, Washington, and Texas. At Lackland, it raced through the military community, striking 106 basic trainees—5 of whom ended up in the intensive care unit. For a few months, it looked like adenovirus 14 might have the makings of a murderous epidemic; in the end, it caused the deaths of 10 people but then petered out quickly. What made the virus such a nasty bug? And what stopped it from becoming the transmissible monster it first appeared to be?

The answers lie in the devil's bargain every virus makes. The bargain is a kind of evolutionary handshake between virulence (the ability to make lots of offspring) and transmission (the ability to spread). You would think being very virulent, making a whole slew of offspring to overwhelm a host, might be just the ticket to perpetuating a viral line. But if you think about it, someone prostrate with aches and fever is not much good at infecting other people and creating new hosts for a cold virus. So a virus has to balance the harm it does its host against its chances of spreading. Just where the balance tips is determined in part by how a virus is transmitted. Like other cold viruses, adenovirus usually spreads with some difficulty through air or direct contact. So it would seem to require a relatively healthy host (one able to cough, sneeze, and spread mucus among others) to help it get around, which would select against virulence. However, the kind of environment offered by a military barracks like Lackland—close quarters, where hosts have prolonged contact and bugs are easily transmitted from body to body without much host movement—can tip the balance the other way, fostering the emergence of a more virulent strain, such as adenovirus 14.

The bug didn't cause an epidemic because this virulent strain couldn't spread easily outside its cozy military habitat. And once the Air Force officials grasped the situation, they put in place measures to reduce the threat—more hand washing, sanitization, and isolation of patients with the bug—all of which not only helped to halt the transmission of the virus but probably also promoted the evolution of a less-virulent strain.

The Centers for Disease Control and Prevention assures us that mutated viruses such as adenovirus 14 are extremely rare and should not be cause for alarm for most people. A much greater concern is respiratory syncytial virus (RSV), a scrappy, ubiquitous cold bug that infects almost all children by their second birthday. RSV may evoke only a mild cold in adults but in babies can trigger acute bronchiolitis—the most common reason for hospitalization of small infants in developed countries. In the United States, it strikes about 45 of 1,000 babies each year, causing 120,000 hospitalizations. The same is true for human metapneumovirus (HMPV), a recently identified culprit in respiratory illnesses. Catch HMPV, and you may get a simple cold, or you may end up on a ventilator.

Still less comforting is the recent news that even more benign bugs, such as rhinoviruses, can act as perpetrators of serious disease. If a rhinovirus infection develops into bad sinusitis or a serious bacterial ear infection, it may cause potentially lethal complications, such as a brain abscess or meningitis. Moreover, with the new molecular detection techniques now used in hospitals, doctors have discovered that the not-so-innocent rhinoviruses land more children in the hospital than does RSV—mostly tots with asthma.

For those who have never suffered an asthma attack, it's hard to imagine the distress it causes. Asthma inflames and narrows the small airways in the lung, called bronchi, impeding the passage of air, causing coughing, wheezing, and breathlessness—hence the origin of the term from the Greek word for "panting." The inflammation makes the airways swollen and hypersensitive, so they react to innocuous substances breathed in with air. Cells lining the bronchi may secrete more mucus than usual, further narrowing the airways. An asthma attack arrives like a squall, squeezing the airways and causing a desperate fight for breath. There is no troublesome or dangerous complaint more unpleasant than this one, wrote Seneca in the first century AD, which "is hardly surprising, is it, when you consider that with anything else you're merely ill, while with this, you're constantly at your last gasp? This is why doctors have nicknamed it 'rehearsing death,' since sooner or later the breath does just what it has been trying to do all those times."

In this country, more than 34 million adults have asthma, as do some 10 million children. Anyone with asthma knows the peril of catching a cold. Some 80 to 100 percent of acute wheezing attacks in infants and young children and around 75 percent in adults are triggered by respiratory viruses. In two-thirds of cases, rhinoviruses are at fault. "Viral infections trigger the vast majority of asthma attacks in school-age children," says Sebastian Johnston, an expert on respiratory disease at Imperial College London. Admissions to hospitals because of asthma attacks correspond to the peak of rhinovirus infections in early fall each year as children return to school.

"People with asthma are more susceptible to these infections," says Johnston, "and when they're infected, they get much more severe symptoms than normal people do, especially in the lower respiratory tract. We're trying to understand why."

The son of a general practitioner and a father of six (who rarely gets colds), Johnston studied virology with David Tyrrell at the Common Cold Unit in the late 1980s, just before it closed. Now his office is on the third floor of the University School of Medicine on the St. Mary's campus in West London. In 2008, in a basement laboratory of the building, Johnston and his colleagues created the first animal model of the common cold, a mouse genetically engineered to catch human rhinoviruses, part of an ark of such "humanized" mice manipulated to express human genes so they may serve as lab models for human disease.

Until Johnston's engineered "mouse that sniffled," attempts to develop small-animal models of rhinovirus infection had failed because the virus won't bind with any nonhuman, non-chimp animal cells. "This has been a major obstacle to the discovery of treatments in the last 50 years," says Johnston. "The mouse model makes studying cause and effect much easier, so we can use it to better understand the mechanism of rhinovirus infection and also how to treat it."

Johnston's main interest is finding an effective treatment for people who suffer severe attacks of asthma and chronic obstructive pulmonary disease (COPD) in response to colds. "In most of us, rhinovirus infection is a mere annoyance," he says, "but in these people, it sends them to the hospital and can even kill them." COPD is nearly always caused by smoking and is noteworthy for the chronic "smoker's cough" it produces, along with shortness of breath and wheezing. In the United States, the disease affects some 24 million people and is the fourth leading cause of death. Exacerbations were once believed to be triggered mostly by bacterial infections, but recent evidence shows that cold viruses are a common trigger.

The reason people with asthma and COPD may end up in the hospital from a cold virus while the rest of us suffer only minor symptoms, Johnston believes, lies in the secret workings of our immune systems. He and his team recently made an intriguing discovery: rhinoviruses in lung cells from people with asthma replicate at a much faster rate than they do in lung cells from people without the condition. "If you take cells from the bronchial tubes of normal people and infect them with human rhinovirus in culture," Johnston explains, "a little replication occurs. If you take cells from the bronchial tubes of asthmatic people and infect them with the same dose of rhinovirus, they replicate a lot."

This was a revelation. It was once thought that rhinoviruses didn't propagate at all in cells of the lung and lower airways because the temperature there was too warm. Now it appears that while the temperature of the lower airways may be higher than in the nose and throat, it is nonetheless just fine for replication. But normally, the body prevents the virus from taking hold in the lower airways.

Not in people with asthma.

Here's where the mouse comes in. To understand how cold viruses spark attacks in asthmatics, Johnston and his team created a mouse model of the interaction. First they bred that transgenic strain of mouse harboring a gene that makes the human ICAM-1 receptor—the little key that allows rhinoviruses entry into cells—thereby producing a mouse that could actually become infected with a human cold virus. Then they exposed the cold-prone mice to both the rhinovirus and to an allergen that triggers an allergic response in their airways, generating a model of a human rhinovirus-induced asthma attack.

Another member of Johnston's mouse-model team, Nathan

Bartlett, leads me to the basement laboratory to take a peek at the famous rodents. At the time, Bartlett is suffering from a serious head cold ("not from careless handling of rhinovirus," he assures me, "just a late-night party"). He stays outside while I suit up in booties and a hairnet and then step into the isolated laboratory. The technician directs me to a single cage holding a male, a pregnant female, and five pups, all genetically engineered to possess the human receptor that allows them to catch colds.

I was hoping for a glimpse of Stuart Little sneezing. But "alas, mice have no sneeze reflex," Bartlett tells me. "They don't get overtly ill, but they show similar changes in the way their airways and lungs function."

"The mice don't have colds quite the way humans do," Johnston confirms. "But we do see the same or similar inflammatory responses—production of cytokines—and antiviral responses." They make mucus just as we do. And in the mice that act as asthma models, there's a worsening of asthmatic responses, says Johnston, "more airway hyper-responsiveness, a narrowing of the airways with exposure to irritants—a cardinal feature of asthmatics. So we can use this model to assess the disease itself and the effects of treatment."

As it turns out, rhinoviruses in the lower airways—like those in the nose—don't cause extensive damage to respiratory tissue. They likely create most of their mayhem by aggravating inflammation. The presence of cold viruses in lung cells make the cells spew out quantities of inflammatory mediators, which fan the flames of inflammation in the airways and make them even more sensitive to allergic triggers.

In Johnston's view, the difference between normal people and asthmatics is this: Most of us banish rhinoviruses from our lower airways before the bugs take hold. We do this with the help of an ingenious mechanism with a strangely unpronounceable name: apoptosis (ah-puh-TOH-sihs), also known as programmed cell death. When lung cells are attacked by the virus, the body normally induces apoptosis in the infected cells—before the virus can replicate and before any inflammatory chemicals are released. The harmless dead cells are then gobbled up by white blood cells called phagocytes. This quick cleanup job is initiated by interferons, the natural antiviral proteins produced in only small quantities by the more cold-susceptible children in the Tucson study. Interferons activate early programmed cell death, thereby aborting the infection. This is the key to a normal, healthy response to the presence of a cold virus in our lungs.

Some people with asthma are clearly deficient in this response, Johnston explains. They don't make normal amounts of interferons, so their infected lung cells fail to undergo apoptosis, and the virus replicates wildly within the infected cells. These infected cells then release hordes of progeny viruses that are free to infect neighboring cells. They also churn out large amounts of proinflammatory chemicals that recruit more asthma-inducing white cells to the lungs. It's a one-two punch that can trigger an acute asthma attack.

A clever experiment revealed the part played by interferons. "If you take cells from the bronchial tubes of asthmatic people and infect them with virus, the virus freely replicates," explains Johnston. "But if you give those bronchial cells a dose of interferon, they become resistant to infection." Interferons are currently available as drugs, but not in an inhaled form, so Johnston is working with his mouse models to develop one—to get the interferon where it's needed: in the bronchial tubes during acute attacks of asthma and COPD.

No one knows why asthmatics have this weird deficiency, says Johnston. Genes likely play into the picture, and environment, too. Johnston has an intriguing theory for the environmental piece of the puzzle.

"Some asthmatics may have immune responses that haven't matured properly because of reduced exposure to pathogens early in life," says Johnston. This is known as the hygiene hypothesis. Like others who hold with this theory, Johnston pins blame for the recent epidemic of asthma on the lack of exposure to a broad range of infectious agents in the first years of life. The idea is that the healthy maturation of the immune system requires exposure to a certain critical mass of germs. "People living in Western communities no longer see cases of diphtheria, whooping cough, mumps, measles, tuberculosis, and many other diseases," he points out. "For the general population, the overall exposure to infection is tiny compared with what it once was. In my view this is why allergies and asthma are so common."

The hygiene hypothesis, first proposed in the late 1980s, has been gaining ground of late in some circles. (Some scientists object to the name, which would seem to scorn good hygiene; they propose renaming it the "microbial exposure hypothesis.") "There's good evidence that high exposure to infectious stimulation early in life matures the immune system and makes people less likely to get asthma and allergy later on," observes Johnston. He ticks off the studies, nearly all of them epidemiological: "Children born on farms, especially those who have contact with animals, are less likely to have asthma and allergies. In fact, on Bavarian farms, where cows are housed on the ground floor of homes and babies have huge exposure to microbes from the mucking shed, asthma and allergy is virtually unknown." And the evidence is not just from rural settings. "Children in day care who have snotty noses all the time for the first three years of life have a 50 percent less risk of later developing allergies or asthma than children who are not in day care," says Johnston, "even after controlling for all other known risk factors, such as family history, breast-feeding, socioeconomic status, etc. Children born into large families are less at risk than only children, and firstborns within large families are twice as likely to have asthma as lastborns."

One intriguing notion put forth by this theory is that frequent and usually mild rhinovirus infections play a critical role in developing effective antiviral defenses, especially during infancy. The idea involves an important concept in immunology. The human immune system has two types of cells known as T helper cells: Th1 and Th2. Both are really good at making cytokines, those little molecules that can inflame or calm other immune cells. Th1 cells make cytokines such as interferon in response to microbes. They also block the production of Th2 cytokines, which are known to be active in allergic disease. Both types of cells are important for our defenses, and a balance of the two is essential for a healthy immune response. The hygiene hypothesis suggests that if a child's immune system doesn't get enough microbial challenges, it makes fewer Th1 cytokines and the Th2 variety runs amok, causing allergic disease.

Infancy is a time of rapid development of the immune system, explains Johnston. "In the fetus, immature immune responses are marked by a preponderance of responses of the Th2 type [probably because these help protect the infant from being attacked by the mother's immune system]. During infancy, these evolve toward a Th1-type [interferon-producing] response. Children with asthma have more Th2-type responses to viral infections. Something has prevented their immune systems from evolving the normal Th1 type, interferon-producing response."

The theory goes that our Th1 system needs exposure to pathogens to fully develop. If it doesn't get this "practice" fighting pathogens, it remains underdeveloped, and the Th2 cells overcompensate, causing powerful overreactions to harmless allergens such as pollen or dander. "Current evidence suggests that the overall load of infectious agents, including cold viruses, encountered early in life is an important factor influencing the shift from Th2 to Th1," says Johnston. When children are exposed early in life to microbes from other children or animals, he argues, the immune system gets the practice it needs, and they develop more tolerance for the irritants that cause allergy and asthma. "I say to all my patients: If it's any consolation, the more snotty noses your kids have, the less likely they are to have asthma later."

Another bit of ammunition for the hygiene hypothesis arises from the effects of antibiotics. Studies show that treatment with oral antibiotics before the age of two is linked with later allergies. There are at least two reasons why this may be: Antibiotics may upset the normal community of bugs living in our guts that are known to be active in shaping our gut-associated immune tissues. Or using antibiotics to kill pathogens may disrupt the normal role they play in maturing our immune system.

Johnston and others are working toward a treatment that may replace the need for actual infection from bugs in the cowshed or day-care center to mature the immune system. "We may be able to find a way to stimulate the immune system with noninfectious stimuli that mimic the recurrent infections experienced by that child in the cowshed," he says. "These would be noninfectious stimuli, such as viral or bacterial 'signatures' that don't cause symptoms but have the same stimulating effect on the immune system."

It is widely believed that the hygiene hypothesis is incomplete or too simplistic an explanation of the role played by infection in asthma and allergies. Like so many attractive theories, this one is marred by some ugly facts. For one thing, allergic diseases abound in plenty of rural, less-than-hygienic environments. Also, it seems to hold true mainly for allergic respiratory diseases such as hay fever and asthma, but not for allergic skin diseases like dermatitis. And here's the rub: some evidence suggests that early infections actually boost the risk of asthma and other allergic diseases in susceptible children. Some scientists wonder if we're imagining the correlation—seeing cause and effect where it doesn't exist—which is not an uncommon hazard of epidemiological studies. "The evidence could be biased," says Birgit Winther. Most of the asthma studies are retrospective—they look back at a child's history after the development of asthma. Bias is often an issue in these kinds of retrospective studies, as opposed to prospective studies, which follow children from infancy for several years to see if they develop asthma. Take for instance the issue of antibiotics. It may be that early use of antibiotics and the incidence of asthma are linked because asthmatic children are more likely to have been treated with antibiotics in early childhood for asthma symptoms masquerading as respiratory infections. In other words, the correlation between respiratory infections in early childhood and the later development of asthma may have nothing to do with the drugs at all.

In correlations such as the link between a child's participation in day care and fewer colds later in life, there could be other variables at play, says Winther. "The higher rate of allergy and asthma among children who did not attend day care could result from exposure to dust mites in the home." Dust mites are notorious allergens. "Not all households are as clean as they might be," says Winther. "Children in day-care centers may have less asthma than those who stay at home because they have less exposure to abundant dust mites. We just don't know the full spectrum of possibilities." In Winther's view, a certain amount of exposure to bacteria and viruses is probably a good thing. "But not too much," she says. "It's a matter of balance."

Chapter 7

TO KILL A COLD

I try all I can to cure it. I try wine, and spirits, and smoking, and snuff in unsparing quantities. I sleep in a damp room, but it does me no good; I come home late o'nights, but do not find any visible amendment! Who shall deliver me from the body of this death?

CHARLES LAMB

The search for a way to cure the common cold has led down many a blind alley and up many a stagnant backwater, but few forays can match the one led by the U.S. Chemical Warfare Service (CWS) in the wake of World War I. On May 22, 1924, *The New York Times* reported that President Calvin Coolidge had sat himself down in a specially designed, airtight chlorine chamber to inhale a mixture of the deadly, acrid gas for almost a full hour.

His purpose? To vanquish the sniffles—a feat reminiscent of the unfortunate effort to treat the Duke of Wellington's deafness by pouring acid in his ear, though with somewhat happier results. (Impatient with his partial hearing in one ear, the Duke called on a quack specialist who tried to cure him by using a syringe to inject into his ear a strong solution of caustic. The acid penetrated the poor Duke's inner ear and destroyed his eardrum, leaving him deaf and in agony.)

The president's physicians were looking for a quick cure for his cold. There was good reason to be fearful: Coolidge had only recently taken the reigns from his predecessor, Warren G. Harding, who had died nine months earlier during a trip west from an infection that began with coldlike symptoms and progressed to bronchial pneumonia. Coolidge was susceptible to severe respiratory infections. A cold he caught as a young man while on a train to Amherst to take his entrance examinations grew so serious that he was forced to return home to Vermont. Moreover, he suffered from asthma, which could be aggravated by colds.

A curative dose of chlorine? Just the thing.

Two months earlier, the CWS had published its discovery of the healing power of chlorine in the *Journal of the American Medical Association*. (It may seem odd that the CWS should be in the curing business, but as the medical journal *Lancet* commented in 1921, "very few people consult a doctor for a common cold, but practically everyone consults a chemist.") Beginning in 1922, the service had gassed hundreds of patients suffering from colds and other respiratory ailments in a small room infused with chlorine vapors. According to the author of the paper, Colonel Edward Vedder of the Edgewood Arsenal, of the 931 people treated—most of them down with the common cold—some 70 percent said they were "cured," meaning that symptoms had "completely disappeared" the following morning, and 23 percent said they were "improved."

The use of chlorine gas to cure the common cold was suggested by observations that men who worked in chlorine plants to manufacture the noxious gas during the war were remarkably free of colds and flu. The same was true of soldiers on the front lines exposed to the pungent, biting fumes of chlorine, compared with those in the rear. A hundred years earlier, physicians had noted that people who worked and lived in the vicinity of bleaching establishments had fewer respiratory infections than others.

Chlorine was thought to act as a kind of thorn-in-the-flesh therapy. Vedder (dubbed "the chemical warrior" by *Time* magazine) proposed that "the irritant action of chlorine stimulates the flow of secretion and cleanses the mucous surfaces," resulting in "productive coughing and blowing of the nose." Through its oxidizing action, the gas was also thought to rid the body of toxins and fuel the activity of white blood cells useful in the attack against offending microbes.

Practically overnight, chlorine therapy became a popular treatment for victims of colds, bronchitis, and whooping cough. In a special chamber near the Senate Appropriations Committee in the Capitol building, the CWS gassed more than 750 people, including 23 senators and 146 representatives. Chlorine chambers in the offices of the Attending Surgeons of the Army and Navy provided treatment for nearly 3,000 members of the military and others. For the general public, there was Chlorine Respirine, 50 treatments for $0.50 in a handy collapsible tube, each dose purported to "knock a cold in three hours."

The chlorine cure for President Coolidge involved a trio of one-hour sessions on consecutive days, offering a healthy dose of rest for the executive and promotion for the industry. Indeed, as one newspaper quipped, "President Coolidge has made the chlorine treatment so fashionable that members of the smart set who haven't sneezed since Christmas are thinking of laying in a supply of germs."

Edward Vedder even proposed prophylactic whiffing of the

gas in public places (properly regulated, of course) to stop the spread of colds and other breathing diseases. "There is every reason for believing that chlorine may be used in schools, theatres, and other places where people congregate, for the purpose of preventing respiratory infections," he wrote. "In any institution that has a ventilating system, chlorine can be introduced in such quantities as to set up the proper concentration in the rooms supplied. This could be so used in schools for an hour, several times a week."

As historian Edmund Russell has pointed out, chlorine therapy worked wonders as an image makeover for a much-maligned weapon of war. But as a miracle cure for the common cold? The medical establishment begged to differ. Vedder's research included no control experiments, and when scientists sought to replicate his work using controls, they found that chlorine brought no more benefit for colds than any other treatment. Said one physician, "The 'large percentage of recoveries within...seven days'...is evidence only of the self-limited character and short duration of most colds." Chlorine was tantamount to other popular treatments of the day—Dover's Powder, Epsom salts, and hot-mustard footbaths—that is, no better than cold remedies of yore.

If you had lived in ancient Rome, you might have relieved your cold by kissing the hairy muzzle of a mouse, in keeping with Pliny's prescription. In colonial America, you might have soaked your feet in cold water in the mode of Thomas Jefferson or pared the rind of an orange very thin, rolled it up inside out, and thrust a roll into each nostril. Or you might have tried William Buchan's suggested cure in *Domestic Medicine* (1772): "Go to bed, hang your hat on the foot of the bed and continue to drink until you can see two hats"—which at the very least would make you insensible to most symptoms.

If you had come down with a cold in 1895, you might have attempted to abort it by "irrigating the nose twice a day with warm water in which a little borax has been placed," as *Scientific American* advised. "No syringe is necessary; but by simply immersing the nose in a basin of water, and making forcible inspiratory and expiratory movements, holding the breath at the epiglottis, the nasal passages may be thoroughly irrigated. Of course, there are advantages in the syringe, which may be preferable from the standpoint of neatness." If you adhered to Grandma's advice, you might grease your nose or guzzle Sir Alexander Fleming's wartime tonic: "a good gulp of hot whiskey at bedtime—it's not very scientific but it works."

As cold expert Jack Gwaltney Jr. once said, treatments of the past are almost as absurd as some used today. These days a hot new remedy for the common cold gets into the papers roughly once a year, only to fizzle in disappointment. Today's miracle cure is tomorrow's laughing stock.

Not long ago I ran across a museum catalog of old cold remedies, and it was a lot of fun to compare it with the new catalog. Fundamentally, cold medicines haven't changed as much as we imagine. In the current cabinet, for example, is Tylenol Cold Multi-Symptom for "fast relief of the worst cold symptoms," which contains an impressive variety of ingredients—pain reliever, cough suppressant, decongestant, and antihistamine. This seems like ultramodernity until you turn to the old catalog and find remedies with almost the same ingredients—painkiller, decongestant, expectorant, etc.—for a good deal less money. Dover's Powder, for instance, was a mixture of ipecacuanha, an expectorant, and opium, a potent painkiller. Over the years, the cocktails have been considerably deluxed up. For a while some cold mixtures even included antibiotics until they were banned in commercial cold products in 1963.

True, today's medicine cabinet has hundreds more options

than we had in the past. But not a single one will prevent a cold or cure it, and there's little evidence that any will shorten its duration. Some may relieve symptoms, such as stopped-up nose or sneezing—though not without side effects.

"We would be much further along now if we had made decisions a little differently in the past," says Birgit Winther. "Way back in the 1950s and '60s, when we started discovering that rhinoviruses caused colds, the leaders at the National Institutes of Health decided that research on the common cold was not important enough for the government to pay for." Over the past 10 years, federal funding has mostly originated from the National Center for Alternative and Complementary Medicine, at a rate of about $700,000 per year—0.002 percent of NIH's total $30 billion annual budget.

"It was decided that it would really be up to private industry to fund this research," says Winther. "And because the research has been guided by industry, the focus has been on antibiotics and antibacterials, with little focus on antivirals. This has resulted in the overuse of antibiotics. We predicted this would cause the development of antibiotic-resistant bacteria, and that has come to pass. Today, children are dying from community-acquired infections with MRSA [methicillin-resistant *Staphylococcus aureus*]."

Antibiotics are chemicals created in the laboratory to target and destroy bacteria. They're useless against cold viruses and do nothing to prevent secondary bacterial infection. Moreover, they can cause serious side effects, such as allergic reactions. "There is no role for antibiotics in the treatment of the common cold," stresses Ron Turner. Still, according to the Centers for Disease Control and Prevention, antibiotics are inappropriately prescribed for colds at the staggering rate of more than 40 million prescriptions a year.

Why?

As one physician puts it, "The general practitioner is like a barmaid in a gin shop, facing overwhelming demand to chemically alter customers' experience of the world." This leads to the overprescribing of all kinds of drugs for adults and children alike, including antibiotics and cough and cold medications.

"In medical school, you're trained to tell parents, 'It's just a virus,' and send them on their way," says pediatrician Tom Ball. "But in practice, you discover that this makes a lot of parents unhappy. So you start offering remedies without evidence. The drug company representatives show up with their decongestants and cough suppressants, and pretty soon, you've convinced yourself that, gee, if the kid has a bad cough and no one's getting any sleep, what's the harm in a safe dose of codeine cough syrup? Even though you know that study after study shows there's no efficacy with cough syrup, it just knocks them out."

This frame of mind may explain why a 2008 survey found that in any week of the year, 1 in 10 children was given an over-the-counter cough and cold medication. This is a disturbing statistic. Recent findings show that these drugs not only have no benefit for children but can also cause serious and potentially life-threatening side effects, such as hives, drowsiness, trouble breathing, and even death. That same year, the FDA recommended that cold and cough medications not be used to treat infants and children under age six.

Most over-the-counter cough and cold formulas are not dangerous for adults if they're taken at recommended doses. Still, Jack Gwaltney Jr. recommends taking single-ingredient medications instead: a nonsteroidal anti-inflammatory drug (NSAID) such as ibuprofen or naproxen to ease cough, malaise, and sore throat; and a first-generation antihistamine (the kind that may make you drowsy), a compound that blocks the action of histamines in the body, to relieve runny nose and sneezing.

It's surprisingly easy to overdo it with the multi-ingredient cold formulas, especially where pain relievers are concerned. Few people read the fine print on drug labels and may not realize, for example, that a dose of Vicks Formula 44 Custom Care contains 650 milligrams of acetaminophen. If you happen to be taking the maximum recommended dose of an acetaminophen product such as Tylenol at the same time, you could get into liver trouble. Some cold medications contain large amounts of sugar and disguised sugars, problematic for diabetics and those on sugar-restricted diets. Others carry nasty side effects. Pseudoephedrine, for instance, the active ingredient in oral decongestants such as Sudafed, constricts blood vessels, but not only in the nose; it can also elevate blood pressure and produce rapid heart rate—especially dangerous for people with heart conditions. If topical decongestants are used for more than about three days, they can cause "rebound" congestion that's worse than the original stuffiness.

Little wonder then that people seek alternatives. We all have "natural" remedies we swear by. Ask 15 people for their favorite one, and you'll get 15 answers. One friend of mine is so convinced that gargling with apple cider vinegar will stave off a cold that if she feels that tickle in the back of her throat, she'll stop at a grocery store, buy a bottle of vinegar, and toss back her head in the parking lot.

Chicken soup has been touted as a cold remedy by grandmothers (including my own) for the past thousand years or so, at least since the 12th century, when the Egyptian Jewish physician and philosopher Moses ben Maimon (Maimonides) recommended it in his writings to cold sufferers as a source of comfort, nourishment, and hydration. "The meat taken should be that of hens or roosters and their broth should also be taken because this sort of fowl has virtue in rectifying corrupted humours."

Recent research hints that chicken soup may be more than just Bobamycin. Not only is it fed to sick children of all cultures for physical and psychological comfort, but it may have real medicinal value. This is possibly due to simple hydration or the flushing of nasal passages by aromatic steaming. Or perhaps it's the presence of a secret ingredient found in chicken soup, cysteine. The amino acid cysteine is known to cleave the bonds found in the proteins that make up mucus, reducing its viscosity, or stickiness, and hence opening up nasal passages.

Stephen Rennard, a pulmonary specialist at the University of Nebraska Medical Center, has another theory. Some time ago, Rennard decided to put the broth to the test. For years his wife had whipped up a batch of her Lithuanian grandmother's chicken soup whenever a cold was circulating in her big family—a savory blend of chicken, onions, sweet potatoes, parsnips, turnips, carrots, celery stems, parsley, salt, and pepper. (See recipe in the Appendix.) "She told me the soup was good for colds," Rennard said. "I've heard that a zillion times. Then I started to think, 'Well, maybe it has some anti-inflammatory value.'" If cold symptoms are caused by the inflammatory response, and chicken soup can dampen inflammation, then perhaps it really does reduce cold symptoms.

In 1993, Rennard conducted an informal laboratory study and submitted the results as an abstract—mostly for amusement's sake. Seven years later, his research, titled "Chicken Soup Inhibits Neutrophil Chemotaxis in Vitro," was published in *Chest*, the peer-reviewed journal of the American College of Chest Physicians. The study aimed to determine if chicken soup would reduce the movement of neutrophils, common white blood cells drawn to sites of infection and active in the inflammatory response. Rennard collected neutrophils from blood donated by healthy volunteers. Then he subjected the cells to several variations of the soup, including just the broth and different combinations of ingredients. Sure enough, he found that chicken soup inhibits the movement of neutrophils. The researchers couldn't pinpoint the components responsible for the effect, but they did learn that broth alone doesn't do the trick; it requires that magic blend of vegetables and chicken that also gives the soup its flavoring. "I think it's the concoction," Rennard said. "While the identity of the biologically active materials is unknown, it seems likely they are water soluble or extractable. Pureed carrots or other vegetables are not recommended as a remedy, while chicken soup is." Homemade chicken soups other than Grandma's were equally effective, as were many canned soups, including Knorr Chicken Flavor Chicken Noodle, Campbell's Home Cookin' Chicken Vegetable, and Lipton Cup A Soup, Chicken Noodle. (In the Acknowledgments section of his paper, Rennard thanks Dr. Irwin Ziment, whose own chicken soup recipe was not tested as a comparator in the study—"there being a limit to which Grandma's soup recipe should be subject.") The enticing kitchenlike aroma from Rennard's lab drew several colleagues, including one who quipped, "It was the only time in my life when I could work in the lab and taste the samples."

Alas, as some experts bent on spoiling the soup theory point out, just because chicken soup elicits changes in immune cells in a petri dish doesn't mean that it actually affects the course of a cold. And as of yet, no one has performed a randomized, double-blind, placebo-controlled study on the benefits of chicken soup in treating infections. Two enthusiastic soup fans from Tel Aviv University feel that such a study is really untenable, as "depriving the control group of chicken soup would, in our opinion, be unethical."

No common cure for the common cold has been better

studied than vitamin C—thanks in part to a quirk in history. At the peak of his career, Linus Pauling won fame for collecting two Nobel prizes, one for chemistry (1954) and the other for peace (1962). Then, late in life, at the age of 70, he turned his spotlight on vitamin C. In his 1970 book *Vitamin C and the Common Cold*, he contended that taking large doses of the vitamin could not only prevent colds but minimize their symptoms. Pauling's prestige gave credence to a theory backed only by anemic evidence. Before his book and since, more than 30 clinical trials involving more than 10,000 people have examined the effects of taking daily vitamin C and have shown that it does not prevent colds and at best only slightly reduces the duration of symptoms. (Even Pauling's own laboratory study concluded that taking high doses of the vitamin daily could cut back the number of symptomatic days by a mere 0.7: from 7.8 to 7.1.) Taking vitamin C won't hold colds at bay—unless you're engaged in extreme physical exercise or exposed to extreme cold. Several studies have shown that for people living in extreme circumstances, such as soldiers, skiers, and marathon runners engaged in endurance exercise or exposed to very cold environments, downing a daily dose of 200 milligrams of C reduces the incidence of colds by half. Despite the volume of studies conducted in the past, the vitamin continues to be scrutinized.

For years, my family's favorite cold "cure" in the supplement category was zinc lozenges—for no very good reason. The mineral is touted as a way to reduce the severity of symptoms and shorten a cold, but the only really consistent effect reported by quality studies is a bitter, medicinal aftertaste. Zinc's calling as a cold remedy began in 1984, when George Eby, a city planner in Texas, became convinced that zinc tablets effectively treated the colds experienced by his three-year-old daughter, Karen. Karen was being treated for leukemia with immunosuppressive chemotherapy, so Eby gave her various supplements to try to boost her immunity. One June, when she came down with a particularly severe cold and was too weak to chew or swallow the zinc tablet her father gave her, she put the tablet under her tongue and let it dissolve. Her cold symptoms allegedly vanished. Impressed, Eby arranged a clinical trial to test the effectiveness of zinc lozenges against colds and found some benefit. Subsequent laboratory studies suggested that zinc might have antiviral and anti-inflammatory effects.

I would like to believe that they do. I would like to believe that there's a reason my family has been loyal to the lozenges despite their foul aftertaste. However, zinc lozenges have lately lost whatever luster they once possessed. When Jack Gwaltney Jr. and his colleagues reviewed the mixed scientific evidence recently, they concluded that the lozenges have yet to show evidence of any therapeutic benefit at all.

This sort of hard data on the ineffectiveness of "natural" cold cures hasn't slowed the industry. Today, the international market for alternative therapies is a $40 billion business. By 2002, cold prevention and "immune-system boosting" was listed as the second most common reason cited for use of complementary and alternative remedies (behind back pain). A third of the U.S. population and from 40 to 70 percent of Europeans use natural remedies to treat colds. The problem with these dietary supplements—vitamins, minerals, herbal remedies, etc.—says Harley Rotbart, is manufacturers can make outlandish claims of health benefits without being held accountable. Unlike medicines, dietary supplements are made and sold without strict government oversight. Manufacturers don't have to document safety or efficacy. There's no minimum standard for manufacturing quality. There's no requirement for standardization of ingredients or dosing. In fact, there's no obligation even to prove that what's on the label is actually in the bottle.

"This is one thing that fascinates me about the common cold," says Ron Turner. "It has exposed our willingness to do crazy things if we think they will help—from gargling with vinegar to steaming. We will experiment on ourselves with things that may do us harm without basis because our anecdotal experience makes us think it will help. It's one thing to try steaming with water from your kitchen kettle. It's another to spend big money—and people do. We're willing to spend big and take risks, all for the sake of easing a mild illness that always goes away on its own."

So do any of the alleged cold remedies actually work?

Scientists are still sorting this out. The literature is packed with clinical trials of these remedies, says Turner, but most are of poor quality. For one thing, the studies tend to be too small. (If benefits are there at all, they're so marginal that you can see them only in trials with large numbers of patients.) Or they're based only on anecdotal reports of benefits, not any real understanding of the remedy's active constituents or proposed mechanism of action. "This means that the studies are not guided by specific hypotheses, so there's a greater risk of an effect being found by chance," Turner explains. "Vague claims of antioxidant activity or improved immune function frequently attributed to herbal remedies are insufficient for optimal design of clinical studies." Some studies are not properly blinded because the distinctive taste or smell of the remedy is hard to mask. Anyone who has sucked on a zinc lozenge knows what he means: the bitter taste is a dead giveaway. Perhaps most important, with herbal remedies, study results often vary widely because the ingredients of the remedies themselves vary.

Take echinacea. Known by gardeners as coneflower, echinacea blossoms look a little like droopy daisies. The Cheyenne used an infusion of the leaves and roots of *Echinacea angustifolia* for relief of sore throat and chewed the roots of *E. pallida* as a cold remedy. The Choctaw used a tincture of the root of *E. purpurea* (thought to be the most potent species) as a cough medicine. Scientists suspect that certain components of echinacea may suppress the secretion of proinflammatory cytokines, though this remains to be proven. A recent review of echinacea studies found that taking the herb won't prevent you from getting a cold but may decrease the duration of symptoms by 1.4 days. This result was more than a little surprising because a number of reliable recent trials on the herb found little or no effect. The problem with this sort of "meta-analysis," which sweeps in a whole range of studies, is not only that the quality of the studies is inconsistent, but so is the kind of echinacea used.

"It's important to remember that echinacea is not just one product," says Turner, whose well-respected study of the herb in 2005 found little benefit. "Not only are there three different species used as herbal medicines, but they're picked from different fields and harvested at different times. Different parts of the plant (root, flowers, leaves, stems) are extracted and prepared in a variety of different ways. All these things have an impact on what's in a given product." At this point, says Turner, so many different kinds of materials are labeled as echinacea that it's impossible to say whether the herb works or doesn't work. One dropper of echinacea differs from the next, even if both are from the same manufacturer. "Maybe there's some form of echinacea out there that has an impact," he says, "but the burden of proof is on the person who wants to sell it." Turner isn't about to conduct another study on an echinacea product until he has been convinced by the manufacturer that it's effective—and why. "I'm not going to flog yet another bunch of volunteers with virus to show that yet another kind of echinacea doesn't work," he says.

Of course, herbal remedies are nothing to sniff at. There's a long tradition of their effective treatment for all kinds of ailments. Some of today's most powerful medicines were developed from willow bark (aspirin), poppies (morphine), ephedra (ephedrine), and foxglove (digitalis). But for now at least, there's scant evidence to support the claims of most hot new herbal or natural cold treatments. This isn't holding back manufacturers from shilling them as God's gift to cold sufferers. And the public, for its part, seems less interested in the outcome of large-scale clinical trials than in anecdotes and testimonials. The homier, the better.

In the fall of 2004, a former second-grade schoolteacher appeared on the *Oprah Winfrey Show*, claiming to have created a "miracle cold buster." As a teacher and mother, the story went, Victoria Knight-McDowell found herself catching one cold after another. Armed with advice of nutritionists and herbalists, she "took to the kitchen" to wage war on the cold, concocting a remedy from herbs, vitamins, electrolytes, and amino acids, which she tried out on family and friends. It doesn't get much homier than this.

Then Knight-McDowell and her Hollywood-scriptwriting husband launched a cheeky advertising campaign for the product they called Airborne, using Victoria herself, some cartoonish germs, and a number of Hollywood celebrities who swore by Airborne's claims. (How could both Kevin Costner *and* Sarah Jessica Parker be wrong?) Ads almost as common as the cold itself appeared on radio and TV shows such as the *Rush Limbaugh Show*, the *Dr. Laura Schlessinger Show*, *Jeopardy!*, and *Wheel of Fortune*. The effervescent Airborne was capable of "fizzing into immediate action." "Take it before entering germy environments, and you're instantly protected." Already have a cold? Airborne "is clinically proven to nip most colds in the bud."

The ads—if not the product itself—worked miracles, and Airborne became the country's number-one natural cold remedy, with sales of $150 million a year.

Then early in 2006, ABC's *Good Morning America* revealed that Airborne's much-flaunted clinical trial was paid for by the company that made it and featured no scientists or doctors. GNG Pharmaceuticals, the group that conducted the test, was just a two-man gig started up and funded by Airborne for the sole purpose of conducting the study. In short, Airborne had no legitimate data to support its claims. Later that year, a consumer brought suit against Airborne for false advertising. David Wilson, a horse trainer from southern California, had purchased the tablets to fend off a cold on a flight to Europe the previous October. He followed the directions closely ("take before entering crowded environments like airplanes, offices, and schools"), but came down with a nasty cold nonetheless. He continued taking the tablets in the hope that they would hasten his recovery. No such luck; his cold was just as severe and hung on just as long as any other cold he had suffered in the past.

Wilson's case resulted in a class-action suit against the company for false claims, led by the watchdog Center for Science in the Public Interest. "Airborne is basically an overpriced, run-of-the-mill vitamin pill that's cleverly but deceptively marketed," said David Schardt, the group's senior nutritionist. (Moreover, at the time the recommended dosage contained excessive amounts of vitamin A, which can be dangerous.) The suit charged that "Airborne is simply another in a long line of 'snake oil' scams that prey on consumer's naïveté and their hope for a simple cure."

Not long after, the Federal Trade Commission hammered

Airborne with its own complaint: "There is no credible evidence that Airborne products, taken as directed, will reduce the severity or duration of colds, or provide any tangible benefit for people who are exposed to germs in crowded places." In 2008, Airborne agreed to refund money to consumers who bought the product as part of a $30 million settlement. The company admitted no wrongdoing, but as a result of the suit, it did reduce the amount of vitamin A in its tablets and toned down its claims. The word "cold" disappeared from its package (along with all references to its GNG clinical trial). These days, Airborne calls itself an "herbal health formula that boosts the immune system"—somewhat ironic given what we now know about the nature of cold symptoms.

Airborne isn't alone in its overblown claims. Dubious declarations and gimmicks are alive and well in cold-remedy marketing, and the public seems as susceptible as they are to the cold itself. The zinc lozenge Cold-EEZE says it's "clinically proven to shorten colds by nearly half," and the homeopathic zinc product Zicam claims to shrink the cycle of a cold by several days. Roger Berkowitz, the big fish at Legal Sea Foods, appears to have bought the Zicam concept hook, line, and sinker. "If you're a little stuffy, come see me," he writes in a blog post. "Eighty percent of the time Zicam will nip it in the bud."

Zicam relied on an advertising campaign featuring an iconic image it believes helps to boost brand awareness: a rhinoceros—"with its large horn and strong presence, a visual reminder of how tough the common cold can be." Matrixx Initiatives, the company that makes Zicam, launched a "Save the Rhino; Not the Rhinovirus" campaign in partnership with wildlife TV host Jack Hanna, a self-described longtime user of Zicam Cold Remedy and an avid rhinoceros conservationist. The hope was that this clever ploy—a sweepstakes for a free African safari with the company donating $1 for each person who enters—would capture the public's attention in a failing economy. Matrixx also offered some high-tech gizmos, including a cold/flu tracker widget for your desktop that provides daily updates on outbreaks of seasonal colds and flus in your area. And for those on the go, the company provided a mobile application used with T-Mobile devices and iPhones, allowing consumers to check cold and flu activity by zip code. On the product's website, users can identify cities currently at high risk (when I last checked, Wichita, Albany, Tampa, Little Rock, and Fresno), presumably to encourage those heading for these plagued metropolises to buy Zicam. (My little city, I was happy to learn, had only a 3 to 8 percent chance of coldliness.)

These marketing gambits seemed to work. In 2008, Matrixx had $40 million in sales from Zicam products. But that was before the FDA advised the public to stop using Zicam nasal gel and nasal swabs because of their association with the loss of the sense of smell in some consumers. The FDA had received 130 reports of people who had experienced anosmia after using Zicam nasal products. Zinc is known to be toxic to the olfactory systems of laboratory animals—and can be so for humans as well. One theory is that the propulsive force of the Zicam gel pump is strong enough to deliver toxic doses of zinc to sensitive nose tissues. A few years earlier, Matrixx had agreed to pay $12 million to settle some 340 lawsuits brought by consumers who claimed the nasal gel had diminished or destroyed their sense of smell. The company admitted no liability but said the settlement was an effort to end litigation. In response to the FDA's action, Matrixx's shares dropped, and the company launched an advertising claim defending its other products as safe and "specially formulated to shorten your colds so you don't just feel better— you ARE better, sooner."

Like many other "natural" cold remedies, COLD-FX purports to prevent colds and shorten their duration. A pill containing a proprietary extract from North American ginseng, COLD-FX originally sailed into the number-one spot on Canada's rankings of best-selling cold and flu remedies with the help of a high-dollar marketing strategy built around testimonials from hockey broadcasters and players. When its maker, Afexa Life Sciences (then known as CV Technologies), tried jumping into the U.S. market in 2006, it created an ad affixed to tray tables on airplanes in the form of a board game, thereby playing not only on the boredom of jet travelers but on their legitimate fear of coming down with something during air travel. It was an effective ploy. A survey of 400 passengers on the flights revealed that more than 80 percent had used their tray tables, seen the ad, remembered the name of the product, and could accurately describe it. Only 7 percent knew about COLD-FX before their flight. Afterward, a whopping 40 percent said they would buy the product in the future. In 2009, the product boasted $47 million in sales and was selected as the official cold and flu remedy of the 2010 Winter Olympics in Vancouver, but so far it has had little success dislodging Airborne from its lucrative spot in the U.S. market.

Unlike with most other natural cold remedies, there are some legs to COLD-FX's claims. Afexa has standardized the product and is putting it through well-designed clinical trials (albeit ones financed by the company). In one study of healthy adults, those who took COLD-FX over four months reported fewer colds, and when they did get colds, they experienced milder symptoms, compared with those taking a placebo. These are encouraging results, but the study was small, and there was no virology to confirm the presence of cold viruses. Preliminary results from a larger clinical trial of 780 healthy seniors in 2008 suggested that those who took COLD-FX over six months had one-third fewer colds—and in this case, the results were confirmed with tests for the presence of virus.

The force behind COLD-FX is Jacqueline Shan, a pharmacologist and physiologist at the University of Alberta. When Shan was a child in communist China, often sick with colds and flu, her grandmother treated her with herbs. "They were bitter tinctures that my grandma added to vegetables, and they tasted horrible," Shan recalls. "When I got older, I was really curious about what was in those tinctures. Herbalists would say it's a secret—a little bit of this, a little bit of that—and then tell you how to cook the herbs. Every time it was a little different. When I was ready to go to school, I thought, 'Who do I want to be? What do I want to do?' I was pretty sure I wanted to study medicine and how drugs work, and I was strongly curious about herbs."

Shan's curiosity led her down a circuitous path, from Shanghai University at age 15, through one doctorate in China, then, in pursuit of a second doctorate, to Canada (where she arrived on Boxing Day with little English and no money), and finally, to the lab of Peter Pang at the University of Alberta. Pang shared Shan's interest in herbal medicine and encouraged her to use biomedical research techniques to explore natural products. After finishing her studies in physiology with Pang, Shan planned to leave Canada, but then the protests and massacre at Tiananmen Square occurred, and she decided to stay put. She and Pang formed a small company and spent 15 years screening natural products, isolating compounds from them, and using technology to measure their immune effects. "We screened dozens of herbs, including echinacea," she says. "We even screened chicken soup. It was a very systematic study." Shan found that ginseng had many different chemicals that affected the immune system—some interfered with its function; some enhanced it. "Ginseng is one of the most well known herbs in China," says Shan, "used mostly to strengthen health and give energy. But when I was little, we couldn't use it often, as it's very expensive."

It took Pang and Shan almost a decade to develop COLD-FX. "We had two things to overcome in making herbal medicine part of mainstream medicine," says Shan. "First, standardization. It goes back to my childhood—you don't know what's inside herbal remedies. Ginseng has thousands of chemicals. Each capsule, each bottle, is not consistent. Second, we had to find a biomedical way to explain how the herbs might affect the immune system."

To address the first issue, the scientists invented the ChemBioPrint process, a tool to identify the chemical profile of natural products and then standardize them. As for the second issue, says Shan, "after 15 years of study, I can fairly confidently say how the molecules in COLD-FX work on specific aspects of the immune system." Shan's research suggests that ginseng stimulates a range of immune factors, including white blood cells and cytokines, and she has pinpointed a possible mechanism for how it does so—through a special family of cell receptors called toll receptors. However, as Ron Turner points out, it's not clear how this relates to viral infections such as colds and flu. COLD-FX doesn't claim to cure the common cold—just to strengthen the immune system. But as we've learned, this can be a double-edged sword. Enhancing the activity of certain cytokines such as interferon (which squelches viral replication) would likely reduce the severity of symptoms. On the other hand, stimulating the production of proinflammatory cytokines might be expected to increase their severity. Demonstrating that a natural product—or any product for that matter—can affect the course of a cold is a challenging task. An herb such as ginseng might seem to raise the levels of a type of immune cell or molecule in the blood.

But are they the right cells and molecules to prevent colds or reduce their severity? Most experts agree that more research is needed. Other studies of COLD-FX are underway, including a trial sponsored by the National Cancer Institute.

If the makers of certain natural cold remedies such as Airborne and Zicam put an excessively sunny spin on their product, it's hardly surprising. Why should we expect truth in cold remedy advertising any more than honesty in parenthood? Maybe the manufacturers really do believe in their own products the way an overappreciative parent believes in the extraordinary talents of her child. Perhaps the expectation of effective performance brings it about: as long as customers believe in a product, it may help them—whether or not it really works.

Never underestimate the power of placebo, says Ron Eccles of the Common Cold Centre at Cardiff University in Wales. When people believe they are receiving treatment, their symptoms often fade miraculously, even if what they're taking is a completely inert substance—a result of the patient's confidence in the medicine or in the physician who prescribes it. This is not to say that the symptoms are "just" a product of the mind, but rather that the mind can produce truly beneficial effects. Placebos can make warts go away and diminish symptoms of asthma, depression, sciatica, and even cancer. One study found that pregnant women who believed they were taking an antiemetic for morning sickness felt less nauseous and their stomachs heaved less. In fact, they had been given a nausea-producing drug, but the placebo effect had negated its impact.

"I'm addicted to placebos," Steven Wright's joke goes. "I could quit but it wouldn't matter."

Placebo can make you feel better even if you aren't actually getting better. The word comes from the Latin for "I shall please" and first appeared in the Middle Ages. Chaucer used it to describe insincere flattery that can nonetheless be consoling. Thomas Jefferson was well aware of the use of placebo by doctors of his time. "One of the most successful physicians I have ever known has assured me that he used more bread pills, drops of colored water, and powders of hickory ashes, than of all other medicines put together," he wrote. At the turn of the century, Richard Cabot of the Harvard Medical School admitted he "was brought up, as I suppose every physician is, to use placebo, bread pills, water subcutaneously, and other devices."

Uncomfortable, invasive, or painful interventions tend to make for greater placebo effects. So do brand names and higher prices. One study reported that a placebo costing $2.50 worked better than one that cost $0.10. Pill size and color can also alter the effect. People find that red or orange pills are stimulating and blue ones have a more sedative or depressant effect. (Except in Italian men, for whom blue pills cause insomnia, according to one study—perhaps, the authors speculate, because of its link with the Sky Blues, the dynamic Azzurri football team.) There's even speculation that the linguistic aspects of drug names are influential, for instance, "Viagra," with its echo of words such as "vigor" and "Niagara." It's all about expectations of benefit.

Treatments for the common cold are no exception. As early as 1933, Harold Diehl, dean of the University of Minnesota Medical School, gave inert lactose tablets as "cold remedies" to 35 students with acute colds, and they reported being promptly freed of their cold woes. Since then, researchers have noted that people taking placebo in the early stages of a cold experience milder symptoms. Recently, Eccles and his team at the Common Cold Centre found that the placebo effect was a major component of any cough treatment.

Experts believe that the sporadic positive results in studies of some alternative remedies may be chalked up to the placebo effect. "It's at work with any remedy or treatment," says Jack Gwaltney Jr. "I could go out and grind up the periwinkle in my yard and put it into capsules, and if someone believed it would have an effect, it might." Just as warts can be ordered off the skin by belief in treatment, cold symptoms can be dampened or palliated by confidence in a cold product. This may come about through experience. The first time you try a product on a cold, the cold goes away, as colds do—though maybe this one by chance goes away more quickly than most colds. Overnight, you're converted. Even the skeptical, the discerning, become believers. "Often there is this perception after taking something that you got better faster," says Ron Turner. "The truth is, no matter what you do, you'll get better. But in the end, it may be that your faith in a product really does speed recovery."

There's no question that placebo works, but *how* it works has mystified physicians for decades. New research suggests that certain placebo effects may result from release in the brain of natural painkillers known as endogenous opiates, generated when the brain expects relief. Block the action of these opiates, and the effect disappears. In the case of colds, it may be that some similar intelligence or other in our minds knows how to calm the agitated immune cells that generate our symptoms—or at least ignore their frantic messages.

Belief in the beneficial nature of the treatment is essential. So maybe people's disinterest in clinical trials and other scientific evidence is self-serving. I'll admit that for a long time, some part of me didn't want to know about the shaky clinical evidence on zinc: I didn't want to ruin my placebo effect.

There's another dimension to this. If it's true that a dozen different people have a dozen different cures for the common cold, perhaps we should take this at face value. Perhaps different things really do work for different people. If a remedy helps one person and not another, this may be due to a mix of subtle factors, not the least of which is belief.

Why haven't we invented a vaccine or an effective antiviral drug to knock the socks off cold viruses? It's a fair question. We've made great progress grasping the secret life of the common cold, but the sad truth is that we're as stymied as ever by how to cure it.

A cure for the cold is a hard mark for two reasons, explains Ron Turner. First, there's the biological. Because so many different viruses cause the cold, it presents an elusive and moving target. A vaccine or drug that works against one virus or strain of viruses is largely ineffective against the others. Cold viruses are error-prone when they replicate, so they "drift" genetically. Not only has this process produced hundreds of different strains of cold viruses, but the strains can combine to form new ones. When scientists cracked the genetic codes for rhinoviruses in 2009, they found that some of the strains likely arose from the swapping of genetic material between two different varieties infecting the same person. This sort of genetic recombination—once thought impossible—means that the viruses are even more hoppity targets than we ever imagined.

Then there's the practical aspect. Colds are mild and self-limiting, so therapy has to work very quickly to be effective, says Ron Turner. And it has to be cheap. Drug developers say people are not likely to be willing to pay for expensive drugs to treat a minor annoyance like the common cold. But the typical cost of developing a new drug starts at around $800 million. "Moreover," adds Turner, "it has to be absolutely safe. There's no tolerance for side effects. All of this makes for a stiff challenge."

It wasn't supposed to be like this. The strides made during the revolution in molecular biology made a cure seem highly promising. Once researchers deciphered the molecular structures of human rhinoviruses in 1985 and found the little handle they use to attach to human cells, for instance, it seemed a simple matter of finding an antiviral drug that would interfere with the hook-and-eye mechanism. But it turns out that things are a lot more complicated than that.

There are such drugs in the pipeline, known as capsid-binding agents. They're designed to fasten on to rhinoviruses and prevent the hooking from happening. One of these compounds, tremacamra, showed small but significant effects on reducing symptoms when tested. However, drugs were never developed, because tremacamra wasn't effective if taken more than 12 hours after the start of infection, and people tend to become aware of infection at about 16 hours after it has begun. Also, tremacamra had to be taken six times a day, an intolerable inconvenience for most people. The drug pleconaril made more progress—the first such agent actually submitted for approval to the FDA—but then had the rug yanked from under it. In people treated within 36 hours of the onset of symptoms, pleconaril shortened colds by 1 to 1.5 days. This may seem like a modest effect, but some experts anticipated huge economic benefits in terms of recouping lost productivity due to sick leave. However, pleconaril was shot down for safety reasons: subsequent studies showed that the drug disrupted the effects of birth-control pills. "So you don't get a cold," says Ron Turner, "but you do get pregnant—not a tradeoff most women are willing to make."

Another class of drugs, the 3C protease inhibitors, is designed to block replication of rhinoviruses once they've penetrated your nasal cells. Though initial results were promising in experimental trials of one such agent, rupintrivir, the compound turned out not to be effective in natural infection studies.

For more than a decade, Jack Gwaltney Jr. worked on devising a drug that delivered a one-two punch to colds by combining two features: an antiviral (in the form of interferon) and an anti-inflammatory. You need to have both, he explains: the interferon to combat the virus, not because it's destructive—it isn't—but because it prolongs the immune response, like a thorn under the saddle of a bucking horse; and the anti-inflammatory to reduce the body's inflammatory responses. In trials, the drug showed good results, at least for rhinoviruses. But Gwaltney ran into an economic brick wall. The patent on the process for making interferon by genetic engineering is held by a company that uses the antiviral to produce a drug for treating hepatitis C. A tiny vial of interferon costs upwards of $80, making it prohibitively expensive. People—and more to the point, drug companies—are willing to pay only so much.

Researchers have not given up. Among the latest prospects are small interfering RNAs (siRNAs). These are naturally occurring molecules that are capable of silencing genes. Scientists are working on ways of using siRNAs to turn off viral genes in all kinds of infectious agents, including RSV, but we're still a long way from viable drugs. There are also drugs on the horizon, such as the nasal spray tested in the University of Virginia study, based on small molecules that our white blood cells naturally produce, which are designed to nip viral activity in the bud. But again, it will be some time before they find their way onto market shelves.

Another new prospect grows out of our understanding that cold symptoms result from the body's inflammatory response to the presence of the cold virus. This suggests the possibility of treating a cold by "normalizing" how the body responds to viruses. Scientists are looking for molecules that might affect the immune system in this way. Vitamin D has been proposed as a candidate, though the research is preliminary, and much work remains to be done to confirm its efficacy.

A promising possibility for a vaccine against rhinoviruses has emerged of late. Some scientists suspect that the many various strains of rhinovirus may all share certain conserved bits of viral protein in their outer coats. Unlike other outer-coat proteins, these don't change as the virus replicates. These stable, shared protein pieces could serve as antigens, or flags, for broad-spectrum vaccines effective against the 100-plus strains of rhinovirus. However, says Ron Turner, it's going to be a long time before we have a working vaccine in hand. "I don't think I'm going to be out of a job anytime soon."

At the moment, it seems, by faith alone can man truly stave off or shorten his cold.

Or perhaps there is another way. One new study suggests that simple empathy is about as effective as potent drugs such as pleconaril in treating colds, cutting short a cold by one whole day. No joke. In 2009, researchers found that if cold sufferers feel their doctor is truly empathetic—friendly, reassuring, making them feel at ease, allowing them to tell their own story, really listening, understanding their concerns, showing care and compassion, and helping them plan a course of action—their cold is reduced by a full day compared with patients who do not get this warm and fuzzy bedside treatment. Moreover, the treatment requires only a single dose and has no side effects. Of course a single study does not conclusive evidence make. But what's the harm? For now, perhaps it's prudent to follow writer Robert Benchley's advice: "If you think that you have caught a cold, call in a good doctor." Better yet, "Call in three good doctors and play bridge."

Chapter 8

DON'T CATCH ME IF YOU CAN

Might we have better luck avoiding colds in the first place?

My friend Cathy carries those little bottles of Purell everywhere she goes. She has them in her purse and her computer bag, in her desk drawers and her car. She uses them after she shakes hands with anyone or goes into a store, particularly a pharmacy. She never opens a door with her bare hands but uses her sweater or a shirt. She flushes toilets with her foot, presses elevator buttons with her elbow. If she is seated in a plane next to someone with a cough, she says, "It totally freaks me out. I do everything I can to move. Even it if means creating a story like, I have cancer and can't be near a sick person. Yes, I did use that one," she admits. "If I absolutely *have* to stay there, I try not to talk and keep my face averted. Afterwards, I take vitamin C."

Cathy's pediatrician father put the fear of germs in her. At parties, he instructed his children on which guests to avoid kissing and which to stay away from altogether. Her mother's constant refrain was "Keep your fingers away from your face. Don't put your fingers in your mouth!" "As a result, I pretty much see the world with an overlay of little floating germs," she says, "and my goal is to avoid them in every way possible." In the past 12 years, Cathy hasn't had a single cold. But at what cost? "Before I go on vacation, I won't go anywhere or see anyone except my fiancé," she says. "And I definitely won't go to a movie theater or any other place where there are lots of people, or, God forbid, kids. I love kids, but they make me really nervous on the germ front. My cousins have gotten used to my asking if they are sick before I commit to coming over to their house; they completely understand now when I back out."

Cathy is in famously good company. Marcel Proust, Marlene Dietrich, and Howard Hughes were germaphobes. Cameron Diaz opens doors with her elbows. Jessica Alba of *Fantastic Four* fame reportedly carries a UV light to zap germs in her hotel rooms. Donald Trump considers shaking hands "barbaric"—an aversion that got him in hot water with the unwashed masses during his 2000 presidential campaign. "People always come up to me wanting to shake hands and I never know where that hand has been," he writes in his blog. "I say let's copy the wonderful Japanese custom of bowing. It's respectful and it's sanitary." Trump's campaign reportedly handed out half-ounce bottles of hand sanitizer to his constituents (tagged with his website address). The comedian Howie Mandel, who once wowed his audiences by blowing up a surgical glove using only his nose, fist-bumps acquaintances instead of shaking hands to avoid germs. The jacket of his new book, *Don't Touch Me*, shows Mandel inside a man-size plastic bubble; his website sells blue wristbands reading "Skip the Shake." Word has it that he even built a special guesthouse that he could retreat to when his kids got sick.

Our society as a whole is far more germ conscious than it was, say, 10 or 15 years ago, says Harley Rotbart. "This is in part because we're inundated with news stories about health and infection. The types of stories that a decade ago might not have made the newspaper are now breaking news on all of the cable channels. When there are five cases of peanut butter associated with salmonella or two cases of *E. coli* linked with spinach, it becomes a huge national story and people wonder whether they should be eating spinach or peanut butter," says Rotbart. "But," he adds, "there's also clearly a sales job going on here." The enterprising germ-fighting industry exploits our fears, flooding the market with antimicrobial lotions, soaps, shampoos, toothpaste, perfume, air fresheners. You can buy hundreds of products infused with the antimicrobial chemical triclosan (the antibiotic present in most antibacterial soaps), including pencils and protractors for children. This is a complete scam, says Rotbart. "How can anyone believe that an antibiotic embedded in plastic can kill a bug that lands on the surface of an object? I understand the economics of it but not the biology. A plain protractor costs $0.35 and one impregnated with antibiotic costs $1.50. But how does an antimicrobial in a protractor or a hairbrush or a toilet seat find the bacteria it's supposed to destroy? This is the sort of nonsense that preys on the paranoia of people prone to paranoia."

The kind of hypervigilance that has come to characterize our culture may have some subtle psychological effects. Rotbart doesn't worry too much about its impact on children—he believes they're resilient and won't succumb to obsession over cleanliness. But at least one study suggests that even educated adults are affected by the germ hype in unexpected ways, making us overreact to something as simple as a sneeze. The study, led by Spike Wing Sing Lee of the University of Michigan, suggests that awareness of the danger of infectious disease heightens our perception of risks posed by other, unrelated hazards. Last May, just when swine flu was beginning to emerge as a serious threat, Lee and his colleagues positioned an actor in a busy building on the Michigan campus. As students passed, the actor occasionally sneezed loudly. Then the psychologists waylaid the students and interviewed them. Those who had witnessed the sneeze perceived a greater risk not only of getting sick but also of risks utterly unrelated to germs—such as having a heart attack before age 50 or dying in an accident or as a result of a violent crime. When asked about their views on this country's health-care system (was it a disaster or working pretty much okay?), the sneeze perceivers tended to pan the current system and express the view that resources should be shifted from the creation of green jobs to vaccine development.

In other words, in an atmosphere of hypervigilance, a simple sneeze can trigger sweeping fears and even color people's views on something as abstract as government allocation of resources.

"It's hard not to be conscious of germs when there's a hand sanitizer dispenser outside every classroom and in every public bathroom," says Rotbart. "We're a Purell-inundated society." In Rotbart's view, this is not necessarily a bad thing. For starters, it means that people who are sick are generally more aware that they may be contagious and thus take more precautions. "More often these days, you hear people with a cold saying, 'Hey, you don't want to shake my hand; let's do an elbow bump instead.' It's not necessarily that the potential recipients of a bug are more paranoid, it's that the 'donors' have become more conscientious."

Rotbart advocates what he calls "prudent paranoia": being careful about those things that present a real risk and chilling out about those things that don't. "We don't need to worry about every handrail or doorknob or elevator button or computer keyboard," says Rotbart. "We don't need to raise our children in a society where every shopping cart goes through a car wash. Telling our kids they have to wash their hands every time they play with a playmate is just goofy," says Rotbart. "But telling them to charge into the dugout and get a squirt of hand sanitizer before they eat those quartered oranges with their fingers after they've just high-fived the 25 members of the opposing baseball team in the middle of the cold or flu season—that's just smart."

There is really only one surefire way to escape cold bugs altogether: become a hermit. Second best: stay away from children.

Short of these somewhat impractical steps?

Scientists are deeply interested in the question, as it may have some bearing on stopping the spread of pandemic flu. The Centers for Disease Control and Prevention has funded a series of international projects probing the best preventive strategies, among them a project known affectionately as the STUFFY Trial—or Stopping Upper Respiratory Infections and Flu in the Family—directed by Elaine Larson of the Columbia University School of Nursing. Larson has been studying the effect of face masks, hygiene, and other methods in preventing the spread of colds and flu in 450 mostly Hispanic households in northern Manhattan.

Where colds are concerned, masks appear to be of little value. They're inconvenient, so it's difficult to get people to wear them, says Larson. To encourage compliance with children, Larson's team used pediatric masks with Winnie the Pooh on them. But getting a two-year-old to keep a face mask on—even one with a fat, smiling bear on the front—is nearly impossible. In any case, as Larson points out, masks are unlikely to catch on here because they're not culturally acceptable in this country the way they are in Asia. Even in Asia, however, where they're commonly worn to prevent respiratory infections, they're not much good against colds, according to recent studies in Hong Kong and Japan. (Although, as the Japanese authors concluded somewhat opaquely, "a larger study is needed to definitively establish noninferiority of no mask use.")

Jack Gwaltney Jr. suggests that face masks may be useful in fighting pandemic flu, however—"as long as they cover eyes and nose, and they're worn 24 hours a day for three months."

Given the churning concern over swine flu in 2009, it's perhaps not surprising that the year's Ig Nobel winner in the Public Health category was the inventor of a face mask—well, a bra—well, a bra that "in an emergency, can be converted into a pair of protective face masks, one for the wearer, and one to be given to some needy bystander." This ingenious bit of chest wear was invented by Elena Bodnar, director of the Trauma Risk Management Research Institute in Chicago. To the delight of a packed crowd at the Ig Nobel award ceremony, Bodnar reached inside the top of her dress and pulled out a hot-pink bra. This she quickly disassembled, placing one mask over the blushing face of Paul Krugman, the 2008 Nobel economics laureate. "It takes only 25 seconds [for a woman] to use this protective personal device," said Bodnar. "Five seconds to remove, convert, and put on her own mask and 20 seconds to look around and wonder which lucky man she will save with the second mask."

Really, the best advice for dodging cold bugs may be the simplest, says Elaine Larson: wash your hands, and don't touch your face. If you can adhere to these two rules, you will be well on your way to cold-free dreamland. But this is easier said than done. Just try not touching your face for a day. "People who work on their computers in particular are constantly touching their faces," says Elaine Larson. Most of us do so one to three times every five minutes (200 to 600 times a day). It's a hard habit to beat.

At least if your hands are clean, the risk of passing a virus to your eyes and nose is radically reduced.

The commonsense but lifesaving notion of hand washing we owe to an observant Hungarian doctor who met a tragic end. Ignac Semmelweis worked in the maternity ward of a hospital in Vienna in the 19th century. He was horrified by the alarming rate at which mothers in his ward died from puerperal, or childbed, fever—about one in three, a rate some 5 to 10 times that of women who delivered by midwives at home. The ghastly disease of raging fever, painful abscesses, and sepsis killed its victims within 24 hours of delivery. Semmelweis described the "heart-rending" scenes of women begging to be discharged from his ward because "they believed that the doctor's interference was always the precursor of death." The problem, he concluded, was that doctors and medical students themselves were spreading the deadly infection. The typical medical student and his professor began their day performing autopsies on women who had just died of puerperal fever, then proceeded on their merry way from cadavers to women in labor, with nary a splash in between.

Semmelweis surmised that the fever might be caused by some type of "morbid poison" spread by hand from the dead to the living. He initiated a hand-washing regimen throughout the hospital, insisting that medical students scrub their hands in chlorine antiseptic solution to rid them of the putrid "particles" of the cadavers. Mortality rates fell dramatically, to the same level as with midwives. But Semmelweis's idea was a subversive one, ridiculed by his superior and certain colleagues, who sabotaged his efforts and denied him a promotion—perhaps because of Semmelweis's temper. (Those who crossed him he decried as "partners in this massacre," "medical Neros," and "murderers.") His lack of diplomacy riled the establishment and resulted in his exile from Vienna. At the age of 47, Semmelweis was committed to a mental hospital and died just two weeks later of uncertain cause. Some believe it was from a finger infection he contracted during an autopsy; others suspect he was beaten to death by hospital staff. Despite his unfortunate end, Semmelweis is now regarded as a hero, savior of mothers and father of infection control.

According to the Centers for Disease Control and Prevention, simple hand washing is the single most effective method of preventing the spread of colds and other transmissible diseases. A powerful piece of evidence for this comes from the military. Some 90 percent of all military recruits succumb to respiratory infections in their first few months of basic training. This, in army lingo, "compromises military readiness." So specialists in preventive medicine have explored a range of strategies for controlling infections among recruits. They have tried dust suppression, ultraviolet radiation, disinfectant vapors, mass prophylaxis with antihistamines, and finally, hand washing. In Operation Stop Cough, recruits were instructed to wash their hands at least five times a day. Outpatient visits for respiratory illness fell by almost half.

Most of us know that hand washing helps prevent disease. But not all scrubbings are created equal. Experts suspect that the majority of people don't wash their hands properly. Most flick their fingers under a trickling faucet and consider the job done. Not so fast.

I once participated in a Hand Washing Olympics at a conference on infectious disease in Washington, D.C. Hundreds of people lined up to compete in a test of their powers of personal hygiene. First we rubbed our hands with a globule of cream containing a dye that glows green under ultraviolet light (a surrogate for germs). Then we proceeded on to three separate stations to scrub the stuff off our hands with soap and warm water. At the end, we were invited into a discreet, curtained area to have our hands examined under UV light.

What an embarrassment. My hands looked like a neon Jackson Pollock.

Proper hand washing is a matter not just of frequency and duration but technique. Plain old soap and water do the best job. While ordinary soap doesn't inactivate cold viruses, it does help to dislodge them—but only with 15 to 20 seconds of vigorous rubbing of all surfaces to release the microbes from the skin, including between fingers and under fingernails and jewelry. (Don't scrub too hard, however, as this can damage your skin, resulting in cracks and small cuts that give viruses a place to grow.) If you use bar soap, keep it on a drain stand rather than in a soapy dish. Because soap itself doesn't kill microbes, "germs can live in the soapy goo for a long time," writes Harley Rotbart, "potentially becoming a source for transmitting infections." It's wise to rinse thoroughly, turn off the faucet with a paper towel, and dry your hands with a disposable paper towel. "The dryer your hands, the fewer the transmissible germs to seep onto inanimate surfaces," says Rotbart. If you're in a public bathroom, use a paper towel when opening the door to protect yourself from the last person who left the room without washing hands.

Antibacterial soaps and detergents are useless in the battle against colds. When Elaine Larson took a look at the effects of different kinds of cleaning products in preventing the transmission of colds and flu, she found that all products worked equally well. There was no advantage to the antibacterial soaps and scrubbers touted by manufacturers. That's because of the nature of cold germs—they're viruses, not bacteria. "Any soap or detergent or shampoo that kills 99.9 percent of bacteria doesn't do anything to protect you from the common cold," says Rotbart. "So much of the advertising of these products as offering you additional protection from colds and flu is hyperbole. Washing with soap and water helps, but the antibacterial portion does nothing to add protection."

In fact, antibacterial soaps aren't all that effective at fighting bacteria either. One study showed that people who washed with antibacterial soap for a year had the same bacteria count on their hands as people who washed with plain soap. The active ingredient in these soaps is the antibiotic triclosan, which doesn't kill many bacteria but just makes hands a little less hospitable to them. (The study also showed that use of triclosan in antibacterial soaps didn't increase antibiotic resistance, as had been feared—though the agent appears to do so in the laboratory.)

Soap or no soap, how many of us actually wash our hands on a regular basis, especially after activities that would seem to call for it—after bathroom use, sneezing, coughing, and shaking hands; before eating, etc.? Surveys show that most people believe that other people don't wash up as often as they should. They're right.

The American Society for Microbiology has been spying on American hand-washing habits for more than a decade, and their report card reveals some unsettling statistics. Surveys found that while roughly 9 out of 10 people say they wash their hands regularly, only 7 in 10 actually do. Women do a little better than men.

Consider the folks who pass through the nation's airports. How many fail to wash their hands after using public facilities? At New York's JFK Airport, 37 percent of men and 22 percent of women; at O'Hare in Chicago, 38 percent of men and 15 percent of women. Only around one in three adults always washes up after sneezing or coughing in the hands. A 2007 survey by the Soap and Detergent Association revealed that 17 percent of dads report never washing after sneezing. And only around one in four people washes up after shaking someone's hand.

Peer pressure ups the percentages a little. So does the right equipment: People are more likely to wash their hands if they're provided with touch-free soap dispensers rather than manually operated ones. Children are motivated by fragrant beauty soaps in bold colors and shapes.

It also helps to understand how colds spread. Some stubborn misconceptions are still swirling around out there. A 2008 survey conducted by Elaine Larson and her team as part of the STUFFY Trial showed that the majority of adult members in the study's 450 households attributed colds to weather-related conditions, and some 10 percent of respondents blamed evil eye (*mal de ojo*) or sudden fright (*susto*). In conclusion, the authors called for a comprehensive educational campaign.

The government of Great Britain recently launched such an effort. The "Catch it, Bin it, Kill it" campaign began with a giant human sneezing spectacle performed by actors in Trafalgar Square to show that colds are spread by germs—and just how far cold germs from a sneeze may travel when no tissue is in sight. It also included widespread advertising on buses, trains, and tubes reminding people how to avoid spreading germs with the help of disposable tissues and thorough hand washing. To follow up, a "Hanky Amnesty" was declared in supermarkets everywhere, "encouraging shoppers to trade in their old unhygienic handkerchiefs in return for disposable tissues."

A hanky amnesty. There will always be an England.

And a United States. What seems to work in this country is "gross messaging." In 2007, researchers at the University of Denver posted messages in the bathrooms of university residence halls in an effort to get students to wash their hands more often. Promising a cold- or flu-free winter didn't work. What won the students' notice was the idea that they might be walking around with yucky stuff on their fingers if they *didn't* wash. The group tried "you'll get sick" messages, germ messages, and finally "gross" messages containing vivid graphics and photos and messages such as "poo on you, wash your hands" or "you just peed, wash your hands." "We found that the 'gross factor' is what works," says research team member Katie Dunker, "and we were able to increase hand-washing behavior by a lot." The gross messages resulted in a 26 percent boost in hand washing among females and an 8 percent increase among males.

If sink and soap aren't handy, an alcohol-based hand sanitizer is a decent alternative—if you rub it into all surfaces of your hands (between fingers, front, back, etc.). In one laboratory study in 2010, Ron Turner and his team at the University of Virginia found that alcohol hand sanitizers were significantly more effective at removing rhinoviruses than hand washing with soap and water. However, previous studies in natural settings have not found this to be the case, perhaps because people tend to recontaminate their hands after using sanitizer. Still, like my friend Cathy, Elaine Larson always carries a bottle in her purse. "Living in New York City, we come into close contact with a lot of people on the subway, in elevators, etc.," says Larson. "We shouldn't turn into Lady Macbeth, but it's a good idea to keep hand sanitizer with you and use it often."

Alcohol is perhaps the oldest of antiseptic agents. The term is derived from the Arabic *al kuhul*, used by ancient Egyptians to treat eye infections in newborns. Alcohol's germ-busting action comes from its ability to denature, or alter, the proteins in microbes and to dissolve the lipids that make up the envelopes of some viruses. However, hand sanitizers are generally more effective against bacteria than viruses. And they're more effective against flu viruses and RSV, which have lipid envelopes, than against rhinoviruses, which don't. The problem is that a single rhinovirus particle can cause infection, so effective prevention against colds requires complete eradication of the virus, and the 62 percent ethanol content of most hand sanitizers can't achieve that. Moreover, while alcohol may "kill" some viruses, it's effective for only a short time.

Ron Turner is working to develop an antiviral lotion with staying power—in essence, a hand sanitizer made with alcohol and a blend of organic acids that lower the pH on your hands, making them inhospitable to rhinoviruses. In a clinical trial in 2005, he and his team applied the lotion to the fingers of volunteers and let it dry. Then they contaminated the fingers of each volunteer's hand with 100 particles of rhinovirus and asked the volunteers to self-inoculate by picking their noses and rubbing their eyes. The lotion not only zapped the rhinoviruses on contact but remained effective for hours after it was applied. No one got sick. The catch, however, is that the volunteers didn't use their hands between contamination and self-inoculations but sat with them held in the air for four long hours—not an easy task.

Will these lotions stop viruses in the real world, where people are rubbing hands, tapping keys, squeezing phones, and clutching subway rungs?

In the fall of 2008, I joined a group of more than 400 volunteers in a study aimed at finding out. Half of us received bottles full of the antiviral lotion (organic acids in a 62 percent alcohol solution); the other half got bottles of placebo, a lotion with just alcohol solution and no organic acids. We were given several bottles to take home and asked to apply the lotion every four hours and also after washing our hands. We also kept track of any side effects (such as red or irritated hands or eyes) and cold symptoms. Once a week we came in for a nasal wash, which involved receiving a squirt up the nose of saltwater, then blowing the fluid into collection cups to test for the presence of virus. (I rather enjoyed these visits because the nurse had a sense of humor almost as quick as her nasal lavage; the whole thing was over in a snort.) The lotion itself was a little gooey and unpleasant when first applied and seemed to take forever to dry so that I had to sit waving my paws in the air for several minutes before I could touch my keyboard. It did keep my hands moist over the winter when they're usually red and raw from washing. Whether I got the real stuff or the placebo I have no idea, but during the 12-week trial over the peak cold season, I came down with only one mild cold (whereas I typically get the statistical two).

When the results were in, it turned out there was no significant difference in the number of colds contracted by the two groups. "It wasn't that nothing worked," said Turner. "It's that everything worked." Both groups had fewer colds than normal—probably, says Turner, because of the placebo effect: Everyone in the study was more conscious of their hands, washing them more often and keeping them away from nose and eyes (to avoid irritation from the lotion). Still, Turner has high hopes for these virucidal hand treatments and will continue testing them. If they pan out, it will likely require at least another year or two of testing and development before we, the public, get our hands on them.

The other approach to interrupting the spread of colds is disinfecting contaminated surfaces. As we've learned lately, cold viruses have a knack for hanging on to commonly touched surfaces, especially those made of plastic, stainless steel, and other hard, nonporous materials, such as door handles, stair railings, remotes, phones, and light switches. "We still don't know the best way to clean surfaces," says Birgit

Winther. "Wiping them with a damp cloth may just spread the virus around." So Winther is currently pursuing the question: How best to remove cold bugs from surfaces in home and workplace?

One sunny day in July, a volunteer—I'll call her Hattie—comes to Winther's lab to help tease apart the possibilities. Hattie works at the University of Virginia Hospital and is plenty aware of the hazards of dirty surfaces. In the hospital restrooms, "I turn off the spigot with my elbow and close the door with my foot," she says. Nevertheless, the previous fall, she had come down with a roaring cold and took the opportunity to respond to an ad from Winther's lab calling for volunteers: "Do you have a new cold and are you willing to collect a lot of your nasal secretions?" Hattie agreed to harvest a teaspoon of her own mucus within the first 48 hours of the start of her cold ("not much fun," she admits, but worth the cash reward). This she submitted to Winther's lab. The sample was tested for rhinovirus—with positive results—and then stored frozen at –70 degrees Celsius.

Six months later, Hattie is reunited with her cold secretions to test the efficacy of various cleansers. Hattie's the perfect candidate for the job: she won't get a cold from this particular strain of rhinovirus because she already possesses antibodies to it and is therefore immune. (Scientists don't like to make people sick unless they have to.) Winther's team swabs Hattie's mucus across the touch-tone buttons of eight telephones and allows it to dry—"only a tiny bit, a dab," says Winther, as much as might get there by way of a contaminated finger in normal life. Some of the buttons have been treated with various kinds of cleansers (water, alcohol, alcohol with citric acid, a popular disinfectant spray, and disinfectant wipes) before they're smeared with mucus; others are sprayed or wiped afterward. Hattie's job is to offer up her fingertips as trial "dipsticks" to see whether she picks up rhinoviruses from her own mucus smear on the variously treated phone buttons. She presses a button with a finger, then dips that finger into a viral collecting broth that will harvest any virus sticking to it.

Winther's study, like Turner's, is ongoing, and it will be some time before it yields results on the cleaning solution most effective against colds. In the meantime, she says, "When someone in my household is sick, I use whatever I have on hand to wash commonly used surfaces—spray disinfectant or even just water. We really don't know what works best, but I think any kind of thorough washing with a general household cleaner helps to mechanically remove the virus."

Someday we may have surfaces coated with materials that zap viruses on contact. The promise of this new technology arises from the work of John Oxford, a virologist who once worked at the Common Cold Unit. Oxford and his colleagues at Retroscreen Virology, a European research firm, have found that certain nanomaterials—for example, silicon and metal carbide ceramics in the form of particles no bigger than 100 nanometers across—can inactivate close to 100 percent of viruses in less than an hour. "It's early in the research phase," says Robert Lambkin-Williams, managing director of the research group. "We still don't understand how it works. But it's promising as far as coating surfaces, door handles, lift buttons, etc."

Until we have soaps or sprays or coatings honed to make short work of viruses, what's the best method for holding off a cold?

For parents who are always catching their young children's colds, Harley Rotbart has special prevention advice.

- Put a bottle of alcohol hand sanitizer at the door of every room in the house and use it as you enter and leave.

- Mini-quarantine your kids when they are sick. This doesn't mean sealing off their rooms with plastic wrap. Just make sure that their clothes and linens are laundered separately, and use alcohol to disinfect their room surfaces—doorknobs, crib rails, diaper pails—all the places where germs hang out. When you kiss your kids good night, kiss them on the head, and then use alcohol sanitizer on your hands.

For the rest of us:

Take Care of Yourself. "The best advice relates to general good health," says Sunita Vohra, a professor of pediatrics at the University of Alberta. "Eat well (lots of fruits and vegetables), sleep well, and make sure that you're physically active."

Avoid Sick People and Children. "Especially preschool and school-age children," those reservoirs of cold viruses, says Jack Gwaltney Jr.

Wash Your Hands Often and Well. "Wash your hands every time you come into the house," advises Harley Rotbart. Also, after any event that involves a lot of hand contact, such as sports games or business meetings. You may also consider replacing the custom of the handshake with the Japanese practice of *ojigi*, the simple bow from the waist, what Rotbart half-jokingly calls "a brilliant infection prevention strategy."

Keep Your Hands Away from Your Face. "When I'm around someone with a cold," says Birgit Winther, "I'm very aware of my hands and avoid putting them on my face. When my children were small and caught a cold, I would try this for a few days, but after four to five days of taking care of them, I was too exhausted to pay attention; that's when I ended up getting their colds."

Teach Your Kids (and Yourself) Not to Self-Inoculate. The big peak in colds occurs some two weeks after children return to school. They pick up viruses on their hands from contaminated surfaces and move them straight into their systems by putting fingers to nose or eyes; then they bring the bugs home to give to you. One study found that training children not to self-inoculate in this way significantly reduced the incidence of colds. I also rather like Niels Mygind's suggestion that right-handed people train themselves to touch their eyes and nose only with the left hand, using a "clean hand" for this purpose and a "dirty hand" for contact with the surroundings.

If Someone in Your House Is Sick, Strategically Clean Surfaces with disinfectant or alcohol or even just plain water. "Focus on the few things in the house that everyone touches—the refrigerator door, coffee machine, door handles, toilet handles, etc.," says Birgit Winther. "When my husband has a cold, I clean these kinds of surfaces at least once a day. Some people still spray the air with disinfectants, but rhinoviruses don't fly though the air," she says. "We need to focus more on cleaning surfaces." And if you have a cold, be vigilant about washing your hands before you reach for that refrigerator door handle or microwave "start" button. You don't have to worry about reinfecting yourself, as you can't get sick from the same virus twice, but this is good practice for protecting other family members.

When You're Out and About, Be Aware. If you're going to the pediatrician's office, schedule your appointment for early morning. Bring your own toys and reading material. To dodge that bug borne by your fellow athlete at the gym, avoid touching your face while you're working out, and wash your hands with soap and hot water before and after you use the gym and between bouts on exercise equipment. Don't bother wiping down the equipment with a wet towel; that can simply spread germs around.

Cough or Sneeze into a Tissue (and Throw It Away) or into Your Upper Sleeve. For a witty look at proper sleeve-sneezing technique, check out the video "Why Don't We Do It in Our Sleeves?" at www.coughsafe.com.

Be a Good Citizen. Stay at home if you're sick. Up to half of workers surveyed in 2008 said they come to work sick. The chief reason? Because they have no paid sick leave or feel pressure from their employer to be on the job. Presenteeism, the practice of going to work when you should be in bed, costs the American economy up to $150 billion a year; colds and other respiratory infections account for more than 20 percent of this bill. Presenteeism is not a good idea, says Robert Blendon of the Harvard School of Public Health. Sick workers perform below the usual standard and have a negative impact on the work environment. Moreover, they share their germs. "It is far better to stay at home when you're sick," says Elaine Larson. "This is hard for people, I know. But it's really not a good idea to be in the workplace if you're contagious. If you have to go out, stay at least three feet from people. Don't cough into your hand and then offer a handshake." Do your colleagues a favor by holing yourself up in your office. Let coworkers know you're sick so they can keep their distance. If you're an employer, discourage your workers from coming to work if they're ill. Don't punish them for calling in sick, and offer employees a bank of paid time off, which they can use at their discretion. The world will go on without them. That is, unless they're astronauts. On February 21, 1990, the space shuttle *Atlantis* was set for a top-secret military mission to deploy a spy satellite designed to take detailed photos and eavesdrop on communications in the Soviet Union. However, the shuttle didn't blast off until five days later, in part because shuttle crew commander John Creighton came down with a nasty cold and was too congested to fly. Maybe they had learned something from Wally Schirra. But the delay cost NASA a whopping $2.7 million.

Relax. It may not be such a bad thing to catch cold now and again.

Chapter 9

IN DEFENSE OF COLDS

And though a microbe has no heart,
From you, sweet germ, I'll never part.
GEORGE ADE

From the look of it, rhinoviruses and their cold-causing cousins would seem malign mischief makers, bent on disseminating discomfort, to be avoided at all cost. But it is not so. Indeed, a case could be made that colds are part and parcel of the human environment—and possibly even good for it. For one thing, cold viruses are Johnny-come-latelies to a legion of creatures already prowling our insides. We're hardly the pristine places we imagine ourselves to be. We live in a matrix of microbes, and despite the avalanche of antimicrobial mists, sprays, lotions, soaps, and cleaning products on the market, it's impossible to dodge them—indeed, we wouldn't want to. Microbes make up the majority of cells in our own bodies (we don't look more germlike because our human cells are bigger than their microbial ones). Our skin teems with bacteria; our gut swarms with them. Studies show that the average hand harbors around 150 species. (Oddly enough, women's hands have significantly more kinds of bacteria than do men's, which is strange because women report washing their hands more often—but the numbers may have to do with gender differences in skin thickness and acidity, sweat-gland production, and hormones.)

We humans are less like discrete creatures and more like bustling ecosystems, occupied by trillions of mostly harmless microbes that give as good as they get, helping us digest food, regulate our immune systems, and stave off disease. There are viruses, too, sharing our bodies from childhood to old age, causing no harm—or at least only minor annoyances.

Cold viruses are merely joining the crowd. Moreover, they are less interested in our misery than their own perpetuation. Look at things from their point of view. The goal of any virus is not to make us wretched—or to kill us—but to reproduce. For millions of years, cold viruses have studied our cell biology and immunology the hard way to attain a cozy ecological niche in which to replicate, then transmit their own. It's not in their interest to make us sicker than they do. As James Lovelock once said, "An inefficient virus kills its host. A clever virus stays with it." It's to the virus's advantage to mitigate its virulence without compromising its ability to transmit. That is the tightrope it walks. A perfectly adapted virus might have a way of replicating that involves no damage to its host at all. Rhinoviruses are perhaps as close to perfectly adapted as it gets, having attenuated their virulence to the point where their hosts are well enough to be up and about, sharing their runny noses at work and school, facilitating their spread.

Some scientists go so far as to say that our relationship with cold viruses is evolving toward one of symbiosis, beneficial to both parties. Jack Gwaltney Jr. disagrees with this sentiment. "I don't think there's anything good about cold viruses," he told me. "Or I wouldn't have spent 40 years of my life trying to get rid of them."

Really, what could we possibly gain from such a partnership?

Well, respite, for starters. Colds force us to slow down. Much has been made of the interruptive power of the common cold in school, work, and industry. That's only one side to the story. We're such compliant creatures that it takes a cold or worse to jolt us out of our ruts. Maybe it's a good thing to be laid up once in a while, compelled by nature to shift our routine and retreat from everyday pressures. A couple of days at home with the sniffles may, in a sense, be health-giving: the change of pace, the pitcher of water on the bedside table, the chance to sip Mother's Broth (see recipe, page 200) or suck honey cough drops, the opportunity to read more than just a few lines at bedtime, and if you're lucky, the sympathy of a solicitous spouse or friend or doctor, all can have a restorative effect on the body that offsets any hell raised. Think of colds as a kind of safety valve. If somehow we did away with them altogether, who knows? We might experience more stress-related ailments, anxiety, depression, and high blood pressure. Perhaps even more flu.

An intriguing new theory suggests that having a rhinovirus infection may keep the flu at bay—that in fact, during the 2009 H1N1 epidemic, the cold season may have saved lives in France by staving off the epidemic while vaccines were in production. Researchers in France noticed an intriguing pattern in the incidence of the flu in that country. Cases rose in early September then hovered at the same low level until late October, then began to rise again. The delay in the rise, despite similar weather conditions and social behavior, was a mystery. When Jean-Sebastien Casalegno of the National Influenza Centre in Lyon, France, looked at throat swabs, he found that the positive tests for swine flu fell just as those for rhinovirus rose. The same pattern was found in Norway and Sweden: rise in rhinovirus, lull in flu; lull in rhinovirus, rise in flu. It's prudent to question the validity of this sort of epidemiological correlation. But there may be a plausible mechanism to explain it. Some scientists suspect that rhinovirus may block the spread of flu by way of a phenomenon called viral interference: "Once a rhinovirus infection has become established, infected cells start producing interferon and other cytokines, similar to those produced by influenza," write the Swedish researchers. "This immune reaction causes the cells to enter an antiviral state." Previous research has shown that people with rhinovirus infection may be less likely to be infected with other viruses—adenoviruses, coronaviruses, parainfluenza viruses, and influenza viruses. If the rhinovirus in fact delayed the flu pandemic in France and Sweden (and may actually have saved lives), ask the researchers, wouldn't this be a possible approach for controlling the spread of an epidemic? Or for developing a new drug?

These most talented of our parasites may also make us smarter and stronger. Cold viruses instruct us, offering our immune systems safe, natural, on-the-job training vital for the development of robust defenses and possibly even tolerance of harmless substances. It may not be such a good idea to try to shield our children from the normal rounds of snotty noses. And if our body's immune response to the presence of apparently innocuous bugs such as rhinoviruses seems overzealous, we should consider the evolutionary record. Research shows that the inflammatory response is present in vertebrates and invertebrates. That we've hung on to it over eons of evolutionary change suggests that the benefits of overkill may outweigh the disadvantages.

What's more, colds teach us something about ourselves and our individuality. How we respond to their presence—and to the remedies aimed at abolishing them—appears to be at least in part a matter of our singular nature, our inheritance, our experience, our convictions, and our psychology. Maybe the difference between a cold that tweaks like a mouse and one that strikes like a tiger lies in both the genes and the beliefs of the beholder.

Only lately has another positive come to light: the hero's part cold viruses may play in advancing science.

Not long ago, society conducted a raging debate about whether to save or destroy the last stocks of smallpox virus held in highly protected U.S. and Russian laboratories. During the 20th century, smallpox killed more than half a billion people worldwide. Some experts, including the World Health Organization, argued that complete annihilation of the infectious particles would be the only way to ensure that the virus would never be reintroduced. Others worried that destroying all traces of the virus would mean the loss of vital information about how it worked and its effect on the human immune system. In the end, the smallpox virus was granted an eleventh-hour stay of execution by the U.S. Institute of Medicine, which set aside a store for future experimental work.

This would seem a wise choice for any virus. Not long ago, researchers developed a method for using genetically engineered cold viruses to target and destroy cancer cells. In 2009, researchers reported a new gene-therapy approach to treating the deadly lung disease cystic fibrosis using a parainfluenza virus as a delivery mechanism. And that same year, scientists studying AIDS announced that a cold virus had brought the world one step closer to creating a universal HIV vaccine. The researchers had succeeded at binding an essential bit of HIV to the surface of a rhinovirus, then immunized animals with the hybrid, creating a safe mimic of HIV that elicited the production of effective antibodies against a wide array of HIV variants but did not cause AIDS.

Tissues in hand, we await the day when the common cold, long the butt of our resentment, will emerge as the knight that slew the dragons of certain kinds of cancer, AIDS, perhaps even obesity. Preserve these bugs, I say. Who knows what skills and secrets rhinoviruses have yet to cough up?

There's more. Once upon a time, all viruses were thought of as mere genetic parasites, finely honed disease machines. It's true that viral epidemics have posed the most persistent threat to humanity for thousands of years. But now some scientists are shifting their view to embrace viruses as champions of evolution, with a profoundly creative role in shaping life, including our own. "Viruses are the dominant biological entities of the biosphere," writes Luis Villarreal, director of the Center for Virus Research at the University of California, Irvine, "the most dynamic genetic agents on Earth."

The viral world is far bigger than we ever imagined, with something like 100 million different types. It's startling to learn, for instance, that the oceans contain about 10^{31} viral particles—enough, if laid side by side, to span the diameter of the known universe. Most of this viral mass is turning over every day because of ultraviolet irradiation. "Thus, every day in the oceans, virus genomes are regenerated on an astronomical scale," writes Villarreal. The same is true on land. Because of their rapid mutation rate and ability to recombine, viruses have a special knack for inventing new genes and moving them around, an idea offered by Lewis Thomas some years ago: "We live in a dancing matrix of viruses," writes Thomas. "They dart, rather like bees, from organism to organism, from plant to insect to mammal to me and back again…passing around heredity as though at a great party. They may be a mechanism for keeping mutant kinds of DNA in the widest possible circulation."

In the view of Villarreal and a growing number of like-minded scientists, viruses may well be the "unseen creator" that contributed to making us human. It turns out that a good deal of our DNA is derived from viral infection. Geneticists have lately learned that remnants of ancient viral infections reside in the genomes of all living things, including humans. Known as endogenous retroviruses, they make up some 8 percent of our DNA. Evidence suggests that these old viruses played a part in the evolution of the mammalian placenta (which by protecting the fetus and allowing it to mature led to live birth—a stunning development in our ancestral tribe), in the regulation of our genes, and in the ability of our adaptive immune system to respond rapidly to new pathogens. Like it or not, it appears that we're descended not just from apes but from viruses.

I have been trying to think of what the common cold is most like. I think it is most like a distant relative who visits once or twice a year, moves in for a few days (often inconveniently, at the holidays), whose slightly annoying habits agitate you (which you admit is as much your own fault as it is hers), who forces you to retreat to the privacy of your room (where you engage in activities outside your custom, such as sipping soup, reading, and napping), but who also reminds you however grudgingly of your deeper roots and your shared inheritance, and who offers you a little personal education about yourself that may well serve you later. When she finally leaves, you're relieved, happy that life can settle back into its normal routine (which you appreciate a little more for the hiatus), fully aware that it won't be long before she's back for another visit. And—sigh—that you may be the wiser for it.

APPENDIX:
COLD COMFORTS

When in doubt, do Nowt!

GRAHAM WORRALL, FAMILY PRACTITIONER,
QUOTING PROFESSOR PATRICK BYRNE

With no surefire preventive or cure in place, what's a cold sufferer to do?

Some experts would agree with Worrall and Byrne. Do nowt—well, mostly nowt. Chances are excellent that if you take nothing, you'll still recover within around seven days. When pediatrician Tom Ball comes down with a cold, he does "just what my mother did years ago: get rest and drink fluids." But if you're bothered by your symptoms, there are treatments aimed at easing them—as Sir Christopher Andrewes said, "to make you feel better while you're getting better." Treatment may also help to stave off possible complications. If a cold gets too firm a footing, it may evolve into a persistent cough, sinus infection, ear infection, or bronchitis, or trigger an asthma attack.

What follows are suggestions from the experts for several approaches to cold care, some medicinal, some metaphorical.

What the Experts Advise

Cold specialists tend to be skeptical of most popular "multi-symptom" cold medicines on market shelves. "A lot of people take over-the-counter preparations," says Sebastian Johnston. "It's their choice, of course, but these things are not proven more effective than simple aspirin or acetaminophen. I don't waste my money on them." Most of these concoctions contain a blend of ingredients, some of them unnecessary and unproven, and the more ingredients you swallow, the greater your chances of experiencing side effects worse than the cold itself. Also, if you combine these drugs with others (such as aspirin or acetaminophen), you can run the risk of overdose.

Far better to target the individual symptoms that are troubling you with single-ingredient medications. (See Rx for Cold Symptoms on page 171.)

Jack Gwaltney Jr. emphasizes the importance of treatment at the earliest hint of a cold—first, to ease symptoms when they're at their worst (first three days of a cold) and second, to limit the buildup of nasal fluid, which may get blown into the sinuses, leading to sinusitis. The trick is to act rapidly to keep the air passages open. When Gwaltney feels like he's coming down with a cold, he takes two single-ingredient medications every 12 hours until his cold symptoms clear—a nonsteroidal anti-inflammatory drug (NSAID) such as ibuprofen or naproxen to ease cough, malaise, and sore throat, and an antihistamine, a compound that blocks the action of histamines in the body, to relieve runny nose and sneezing. There are two types of antihistamines: the older, so-called first-generation type, such as Benadryl or Chlor-Trimeton, which may make you sleepy; and the newer, nondrowsy antihistamines, such as Claritin or Allegra. Only the older, sedating type works against colds.

Ron Turner uses a topical nasal decongestant (sprays or drops, such as Afrin) to deal with troublesome daytime congestion. Decongestants open the nasal passages by shrinking blood vessels in the membranes of the nose, the primary cause of nasal obstruction. (Chicken soup might help, he says, but it's too much trouble to make, and no one in his family volunteers to make it for him.) For runny nose and scratchy throat at night, Turner takes an older type of sedating antihistamine.

Birgit Winther relies on an NSAID, a single tablet of ibuprofen, or aspirin—and only before bed—to get a good night's sleep. Sebastian Johnson, too, takes only paracetamol (also known as acetaminophen).

No one recommends over-the-counter cough syrups (though the public still seems enthusiastic enough about the potions that they fly off the shelves in cold season). They don't work. Moreover, they can be downright dangerous for children. For these reasons, the American College of Chest Physicians strongly discourages their use. Coughing is part of the body's defenses, so squelching it completely is not a good thing.

As for the usefulness of supplements or herbal alternatives: According to Gwaltney, there's good evidence that zinc and echinacea don't work. The jury is still out on such natural remedies as ginseng and vitamin C. However, if taking a supplement makes you feel like you're suffering less, then go ahead and take it, advises Tom Ball—as long as there are no harmful side effects. "Even 'negative' studies that show no difference between a treatment group and a placebo group have individuals who do respond to a given therapy," says Ball. "While there are a number of explanations for this, one certainly is that individuals respond differently to medications. So when a therapy has essentially no risk of harm, in my view, it's okay to try it." But be a smart consumer. Don't fall for outrageous claims, urges Gwaltney. Look at the studies. And if you're in doubt, ask your doctor.

What about treating children? Parents should consult with a doctor before giving any over-the-counter medicine to infants or young children. According to the U.S. Food and Drug Administration, children younger than age two should not be given any cold or cough medications. The risks are too great for serious side effects, including hives, drowsiness, difficulty breathing, and even death. While the FDA has not completed its review of the safety of these medicines in children 2 through 11 years of age, most experts advise against their use—especially in children under the age of 6. The American College of Pediatricians extends that recommendation to children younger than age 14. Before giving herbal or alternative remedies to children, parents should check with their physician. Most of these treatments have not been well studied in children, so it's important to be very cautious.

And remember this advice from Tom Ball: "As we 'medicalize' natural phenomena like colds, there's one treatment that too often gets lost or forgotten." When parents visit Tom's office to get help for a child down with a cold, he gives them "an Rx for loving."

"I began doing this in order to remind parents that even though I'm not prescribing any 'medicine,' there's actually something they themselves can do for their children," he says. "I've been impressed with how many parents (primarily mothers, of course, since they are usually the ones in the office) are comforted and empowered to be reminded that in addition to nasal suctioning and Tylenol, they have a lot to offer. I see their shoulders relax and the tension drain from their faces. Those of us with loving and caring parents all have a memory of being comforted during viral illness. Call the effect whatever you want—placebo, reduced stress—it's important and, sadly, too often gets lost."

Rx for Cold Symptoms

Sore Throat

A saltwater gargle (½ teaspoon salt dissolved in an 8-ounce glass of warm water) provides temporary relief for sore throat. Because saltwater is more concentrated than the fluids in your throat, osmosis pulls those fluids from the swollen area, reducing swelling, which means less pressure on the nerves and less pain. Sucking on nonmedicated throat lozenges with honey or glycerin may also help. Older children may benefit from a saltwater gargle or sucking on cough drops or hard candy (but be aware of the choking hazard).

Headache, Malaise, or Mild Fever

Analgesics, such as aspirin or acetaminophen, or NSAIDs, such as ibuprofen, can ease head and throat pain. However, there's some evidence that the use of aspirin and acetaminophen may slightly increase nasal symptoms, prolong the shedding of virus from the nose, and lower the production of antibodies.

For children under 6: Nonaspirin pain relievers, such as ibuprofen or acetaminophen, in age-appropriate doses. Acetaminophen is safe for infants older than three months; ibuprofen, for children over one year. Aspirin should not be given to children under 18 because of the risk of Reye's syndrome, a rare but potentially fatal disease. Encourage children to drink clear fluids to prevent dehydration.

Stuffy Nose

Nasal decongestant drops or sprays containing xylometazoline or oxymetazoline are helpful in clearing blocked nasal passages, especially before bed. Decongestants open the nasal passages by constricting blood vessels in the mucous membranes of the nose. Drops and sprays (such as Afrin or Neo-Synephrine) work faster than oral decongestants and have fewer side effects. However, it's not a good idea to use the drops or sprays for more than three days, as they can cause chronic inflammation of the mucous membranes, leading to "rebound" congestion that's worse than the original stuffiness. If congestion lasts longer than a few days, switch to a prescription oral decongestant with pseudoephedrine, such as Sudafed (but consult with your doctor if you have hypertension, heart disease, diabetes, hyperthyroidism, or anxiety, or take other drugs). Oral decongestants containing large doses of pseudoephedrine are now available by prescription only because of the drug's use as an ingredient in the manufacture of methamphetamine. Over-the-counter oral decongestants currently on drugstore shelves, such as Actifed, Sudafed PE, and Tylenol Sinus, contain the somewhat less effective ingredient phenylephrine. Children under the age of 12 should not use nasal decongestants.

Some evidence suggests that a saline nasal rinse or spray, available in drugstores, can provide some relief—and doesn't lead to the rebound effect. It's also safe for children.

Persistent nasal symptoms that do not improve over 7 to 10 days may indicate a bacterial infection. See your doctor.

For children under 6: Young children should not use decongestant nasal sprays or oral decongestants. There's little evidence that they work, and they may cause side effects. Try plain saline nasal drops to loosen mucus and bulb suction—or a gentle nose-blow—to remove it. Drinking clear fluids such as water or juice can help loosen congestion.

Runny Nose and Sneezing

First-generation antihistamines dry nasal secretions, says Gwaltney, reducing runny nose by 30 percent and sneezing by 80 to 90 percent. (Not everyone agrees with this: one review concluded that antihistamines don't ease cold-related sneezing or runny nose to any significant degree.) But because of the risks that come with drowsiness, especially for anyone having difficulty breathing, these antihistamines are not recommended for children and should be used by adults only with caution, preferably at night, when drowsiness is not an issue. The newer, nonsedating "second-generation" antihistamines such as Claritin and Allegra are not effective against cold symptoms.

For children under 6: Some doctors recommend running a cool-mist humidifier to relieve runny nose, but there's little evidence to support its efficacy (see Humidified Air on page 183). If you do go this route, make sure to keep the humidifier free of mold and bacteria by changing the water daily and following cleaning instructions recommended by the manufacturer. Because of the risks associated with soiled humidifiers, some experts recommend that you instead have your child sit in the bathroom and steam with warm water from a shower.

If you're susceptible to sinus infections, it's a good idea to keep your airways clear. Use a decongestant and an old-fashioned antihistamine—and blow your nose only very gently, one nostril at a time, for three or four seconds.

Cough

Remember that coughing can be beneficial, helping to clear mucus, germs, and debris from the airway. So it may not be a good idea to suppress it if you're otherwise healthy. Studies suggest that the most effective treatment for cough due to the common cold is a combination of a first-generation antihistamine (such as Benadryl) and a decongestant. Some people experience relief from sipping on hot drinks and sucking non-medicated lozenges with glycerin or honey. The medicated varieties of cough drops don't work any better and are often more costly.

Don't bother with over-the-counter cough syrups (e.g., Robitussin Maximum Strength, Mucinex DM, and Vicks Formula 44 Cough Relief), which usually contain expectorants or suppressants such as dextromethorphan or codeine. There's no evidence that they relieve cough. Some contain ingredients known to ease coughing but in amounts too small to do any good. And definitely don't use them for children. Cough suppressants can actually worsen respiratory symptoms in children and cause breathing problems; in toddlers younger than age two, they have been associated with fatal overdose.

Coughs associated with colds usually last fewer than three weeks; if yours lingers, see a doctor.

For children under 6: No medications currently available in this country have been shown to effectively treat cough in children, and in some cases, they are downright dangerous. As a result, the American Academy of Pediatrics and other experts strongly advise parents not to give cough and cold medicines to children. Steaming in a warm shower (or in the bathroom with the shower running hot) and sipping warm soup and drinks may help to loosen congestion, relax the airways, and relieve coughing spasms. Raising the head of a child's bed may reduce nighttime congestion and cough and make sleeping more comfortable.

If you're susceptible to bronchitis or chest coughs, avoid smoking. Also, try not to inhale wood smoke from a fire, which can irritate your airways when you have a cold. Call a doctor if you develop a fever, shortness of breath, or severe cough.

Trouble Sleeping

Try taking an analgesic such as acetaminophen or an NSAID such as ibuprofen or naproxen. If congestion is keeping you awake, decongestant nasal drops or sprays can help relieve your blocked nose.

For children under 6: Do not give young children sedating antihistamines. To soothe sore nasal passages, try running a humidifier in a child's bedroom. Direct the mist away from the bed, and be sure to change the water daily and follow cleaning instructions.

For All of the Above

TLC, as prescribed by Tom Ball.

What Do Moms Do?

Not long ago, a team of U.S. scientists interviewed some 300 mothers from different cultural backgrounds about the remedies they used to treat colds in their children. Nearly all of them counted on analgesics for low-grade fever and general malaise. Most also turned to chicken soup and to camphor rubs. Anglo (or European American) moms resorted to fluids and moist heat, such as warm baths, warm compresses, and steaming. African-American mothers relied on chicken soup, camphor rubs, and vitamins and herbal teas. Puerto Rican mothers used camphor rubs, chicken soup, and fluids. And mothers from West Indian–Caribbean countries depended on camphor rubs, chicken soup, and herbal and mint teas (including senna, rosemary, Milo's, garlic, and bush tea).

What Do People Want from a Cold Remedy?

In 2007, University of Wisconsin researcher Bruce Barrett published a study aimed at determining what benefit people expected from a cold remedy, how much they were willing to spend, and how much risk they would accept for a given benefit. His study offered people four scenarios for common cold treatments. Each treatment was to be taken three times a day for the first three days of a cold.

Which would you take?

1. A $0.10 vitamin pill with no significant risk or side effects. Won't reduce length of cold, but might reduce severity of symptoms.
2. A $0.20 lozenge with side effects of bad taste and, occasionally, nausea. Might slightly reduce length of cold as well as severity of symptoms.
3. A $0.50 dropperful of an herbal extract that might taste bad but could possibly reduce length of cold slightly and severity of symptoms.
4. A $2 prescription-only pill with unknown side effects. Reduces duration of cold by 24 hours and alleviates symptoms.

And the winner is…

In Barrett's study, first place went to option #1, a stand-in for vitamin C—with 30 percent of people saying they would take the vitamin whether or not it helped with severity of symptoms. The runner-up was option #3, the herbal extract (a surrogate for echinacea), with 15 percent suggesting they would take the herb regardless of benefit. The bad-tasting lozenge (zinc) and the mysterious prescription pill (pleconaril) tied, with only 5 percent saying they would take the lozenge or drug regardless of benefit.

Overall, people in Barrett's study said that to justify the costs and risks of all the cold remedies, they wanted a 25 to 50 percent reduction in illness. As Barrett points out, none of these treatments offer this level of benefit, yet judging from the $3 billion we spend each year on cold medications, people seem willing to pay anyway.

A Guide to Common and Not-So-Common Cold Remedies

What's Hot and What's Not

If the common cold has taught us anything about ourselves, it's that a lot of us are taken in, says Jack Gwaltney Jr. "This susceptibility is indicative of our eternal optimism—and our gullibility."

Airborne. Sales of Airborne may have rocketed in recent years from $2 million to $150 million, but there's no conclusive evidence that the bubbly blend of vitamins, minerals, and herbs actually prevents one from catching colds or affects the severity or duration of colds. There have been no reputable clinical studies. Some experts suggest that if there's any benefit to Airborne, it may be due to its high vitamin C content, 1,000 milligrams per tablet, which may have a slight drying effect (see Vitamin C on page 187). If that is indeed the case, better to go with the far cheaper option of a straight-up dose of the vitamin, which costs about one-fifteenth the price of an Airborne tablet. As for Airborne's ability to repel germs, that's baloney.

Andrographis. The plant *Andrographis paniculata* (known as king of bitters) grows in Asia and is used in traditional

Indian and Chinese medicine to treat infections and fever. Sometimes called Indian echinacea, it's found in cold remedies such as Kan Jang and Kold Kare (most often with other herbs, such as *Eleutherococcus senticosus,* or Siberian ginseng). Andrographis is all the rage in Europe as a treatment for colds and flu, but there's slim evidence that it works. In the laboratory, it shows some anti-inflammatory activity, and a few clinical studies suggest that it improves cold symptoms a little better than placebo. (Note: Side effects include upset stomach, loss of appetite, vomiting, and hives.)

Antibiotics. Heed the slogan from the Centers for Disease Control and Prevention: "Snort. Sniffle. Sneeze. No antibiotics please!" Antibiotics are powerful drugs that fight infections caused by bacteria, such as strep throat and tuberculosis. They are *not* effective against viral infections, such as colds or flu. Moreover, taking antibiotics when they're not needed can cause harm, triggering gastrointestinal woes and allergic reactions and contributing to the growing problem of antibiotic-resistant bacteria.

Antibiotics are often prescribed for children with ear infections. But studies show that antibiotic treatment results in only a 12 percent chance of improvement but a 20 percent risk of an allergic reaction. The American Academy of Pediatrics recommends an observation period of 48 to 72 hours before prescribing antibiotics to healthy kids ages 2 months to 12 years.

Chicken Soup. Most experts dismiss claims that chicken soup has any real medicinal value. It has been shown to suppress inflammation in the laboratory, but there has never been a clinical trial to test its effect on colds. Still, most of us find it soothing, and it certainly helps with hydration.

Cold-EEZE. These are zinc gluconate lozenges containing 15 to 25 milligrams of zinc. Their maker, the Quigley Corporation, claims that Cold-EEZE lozenges cut in half the length of a cold by interfering with the ability of rhinoviruses to reproduce. However, when Jack Gwaltney Jr. and his colleagues reviewed 14 published studies, they concluded that any beneficial effect of the lozenges has yet to be established.

COLD-FX. Made by the Canadian company Afexa Life Sciences, COLD-FX contains a patented, standardized extract derived from North American ginseng root. (See Ginseng on page 182.) In Canada, where COLD-FX is the top-selling cold remedy, advertisements claim that it "helps reduce the frequency, severity, and duration of cold and flu symptoms by boosting the immune system"; in the United States, they claim only that it "strengthens the immune system." Some relatively well designed studies funded by Afexa show encouraging results for COLD-FX, but there needs to be more research to confirm them. In one study published in the *Canadian Medical Association Journal* in 2005, researchers recruited 323 healthy adults who had caught at least two colds during the cold season the previous year. Half the group took capsules with 400 milligrams per day of COLD-FX; the other half took placebo. Subjects taking COLD-FX had 0.68 colds per person, and those taking placebo, 0.93 colds per person—a reduction of 0.25 colds over the four months. (In addition, the colds experienced by those in the COLD-FX group were milder.) Based on these data, you would need to take the capsules for four months for four years in a row to reduce your average number of colds by one. The recommended dosage (two capsules, or 400 milligrams, a day) for four months would cost about $80, so one has to ask: Is it worth $320 to avoid a single cold?

Most experts agree that it's premature to conclude that

COLD-FX can reduce the incidence or duration of colds. However, it does show evidence of some effect. (There have been no studies involving children, so experts recommend against its use for those under age 12.)

Echinacea. In terms of popularity, the purple coneflower is still the king of herbal remedies for cold sufferers. The leaves, roots, and other parts of the plant are sold as capsules, juices, tinctures, and teas. Studies on the herb abound, and the most reliable, well-conducted ones have lately wilted the herb's cold-fighting reputation. While some research suggests that the leaves and flowers of one species (*E. purpurea*) may have a small effect on reducing cold symptoms, recent, better-designed studies find that the herb does little to shorten colds or relieve symptoms. According to the latest reviews, taking echinacea regularly won't protect you from catching a cold, nor will it reduce the severity or duration of a cold.

Bottom line: experts say save your money. "The evidence is strong that it doesn't work," says Jack Gwaltney Jr. But if you decide to buy echinacea, be a smart consumer; make sure your product actually contains the herb, and go for supplements made from the *E. purpurea* species. Echinacea preparations vary widely in quality, depending on the species, the part of the plant used, and the manufacturing techniques. Herbal products are not regulated by the FDA, so their contents are uncertain. For example, a recent analysis of 59 echinacea products found that almost half contained no traces of the herb. (Note: Echinacea may cause mild side effects, including stomach upset, skin rashes, and increased urination. The herb should be avoided by people with plant allergies or asthma; those with immune-related medical conditions such as rheumatoid arthritis or multiple sclerosis; women who are pregnant or nursing; and young children.)

Emergen-C. Linus Pauling would have loved this powdered drink mix, which contains 1,000 milligrams of vitamin C per dose. The famous chemist and Nobel laureate swore by vitamin C. In his 1970 book *Vitamin C and the Common Cold*, he argued that taking large doses of the vitamin could not only prevent colds but minimize their symptoms. Unfortunately, study after study has naysayed his claim. Taking vitamin C won't take a serious bite out of symptoms. (It does have a mild drying effect on nasal secretions, but Jack Gwaltney Jr. asserts that antihistamines do a better job at this.) (See Vitamin C on page 187.)

Exercise. There's little credence to the theory that exercise moves a cold through the system faster. If you already have a cold, exercising won't reduce the severity or duration of symptoms—nor will it aggravate or extend them. There is some epidemiological evidence that people who exercise regularly have fewer colds than people who are sedentary.

Fluids, Drinking Plenty of. Advice we've heard ad nauseam. The truth is, you can't really flush a cold out of your system by drinking huge amounts of fluids. And there are no controlled clinical studies showing any benefit of maintaining steady fluid intake during a cold. However, drinking normal amounts of water, juice, broth, and other clear fluids can help to loosen congestion and certainly prevents dehydration. Not long ago, a paper in the *British Medical Journal* made a big stink about the risks of overhydrating with colds and flus. While it's true that there are some small theoretical risks linked with excessive fluid intake, this is of little concern for most of us.

Garlic (*Allium sativum*). Garlic has been used for centuries to prevent and treat disease. Lately, it has been touted for its antimicrobial and antiviral effects, and the market for garlic supplements is thriving. However, experts say the evidence for its beneficial effects on colds is scant. A major review in 2009 of randomized controlled trials comparing garlic with placebo found only one relatively well designed trial of 146 subjects. Half the group took a garlic supplement once daily for three months (with 180 milligrams of garlic extract); half took a placebo. The trial reported 65 colds in the placebo group and only 24 in the garlic group. These results seem promising, but they relied only on self-reported episodes of common cold rather than testing for presence of cold viruses—a serious flaw. The reviewers conclude that more studies are needed to support claims of garlic's value in preventing colds.

Ginseng. This herb has been used for thousands of years to boost health and stamina, but only lately has science turned to studying its effects on the common cold. So far, there's only modest evidence that it does any good. Research does suggest that North American ginseng affects parts of the immune system, but it's not clear how this relates to cold infections. (See entry for COLD-FX.) (Note: Ginseng has few side effects. However, it is an anticoagulant, so people taking blood thinners are advised to consult a physician before trying the product. Also, it's not considered safe for women who are pregnant or breast-feeding or for children.)

Honey. Honey mixed with lemon in warm water or tea is a common remedy for soothing a sore throat. One recent study suggested that honey may in fact act as a cough suppressant as effective as dextromethorphan, the ingredient in over-the-counter cough medicines—which is not saying much. When a group of children older than two were given up to 2 teaspoons of honey before bed, the remedy appeared to reduce nighttime coughing and thus improve sleep. But this one study was not well blinded, so it's likely that the placebo effect played some part. (Note: Honey should not be given to children younger than one year because of the risk of infant botulism, a serious form of food poisoning.)

Hot Drinks. Who doesn't crave a cup of sweet, hot tea when down with the sniffles and a sore throat? One small 2007 study at the Common Cold Centre in Cardiff, Wales, tried to pin down whether hot drinks, specifically a hot mug of fruit cordial, had genuinely beneficial effects. The sweet apple and blackberry drinks did seem to make people feel better—but only by subjective measures; the cordials did not improve their breathing. It's likely that the improvements were a result of the placebo effect. Still, if a sweet, hot drink makes you feel better, go for it.

Humidified Air. Cool and warm mists have been used for decades to relieve cold symptoms—based on the theory that dry air can dry out mucous membranes, making a stuffy nose or scratchy throat feel worse, and that by adding moisture to the air, you can ease discomfort. However, clinical trials show little if any benefit. If you decide to use a humidifier anyway, always use the cool-mist models for children, as hot water or steam vaporizers can burn. The cool-mist types are also cheaper to run. Whatever kind of humidifier you use, be sure to change the water daily, and follow the manufacturer's instructions to keep it clean and free of bacteria and mold.

Nasal Irrigation or Nasal Lavage (With or Without a Neti Pot). A little ocean to clear out the nose has long been a popular remedy for cold symptoms. It does nothing to alter the course of the illness but may provide some relief. One 2008 study found that children who rinsed their noses three times a day for three months with a saline nasal wash made from processed Atlantic seawater had less severe cold symptoms than children who were given ordinary cough and cold medicines. University of Michigan researchers have found that nasal washing is more effective than saline sprays for limiting sinus complications from colds. To wash your nose, you can use a simple bulb syringe and a basin. Fill the basin with 2 cups warm water and add ¼ teaspoon of salt. Fill the syringe completely with the water, bend over the sink (do not put your head back), and squeeze the bulb of water into the nostril. Let the solution drain, and repeat with the other nostril. Another method is using a neti pot, a specially designed tool for rinsing nasal cavities, available at most drugstores and health food stores. Follow the manufacturer's instructions.

Probiotics. In the news lately for the role they play in gut health and general immune function, probiotics are live, beneficial microorganisms consumed as dietary supplements (or sometimes present in foods such as yogurt and miso). One study of 600 children in 18 day-care centers in Finland found that children taking probiotics on a daily basis had 17 percent fewer episodes of respiratory infections than children taking placebo. The results of a trial in 2005 suggested that daily treatment with probiotics didn't reduce the incidence of colds but did diminish symptoms compared with people who took placebo. However, the treatment included vitamins and minerals as well as the probiotics. I love the idea that good bugs might protect against bad ones—but these are slim research pickings. It's better to wait until we have more evidence before you shell out cash for these alleged cold-fighting creatures.

Saline Nasal Sprays. Some experts recommend saline nasal sprays to relieve mild congestion and loosen mucus.

They're safe, even for children, and have the advantage of not causing the kind of rebound effect found with some medicated nasal sprays. However, a 1998 trial found that saline sprays have no measurable effect on either the severity of stuffiness or its duration with the common cold—and fewer than half of the subjects in the study said they would use the nasal spray again.

Saltwater Gargle. This age-old remedy, gargling with a solution of ½ teaspoon salt dissolved in an 8-ounce glass of warm water, temporarily relieves sore throat—perhaps by reducing swelling or clearing mucus, which carries those inflammatory mediators that increase the sensitivity of pain receptors.

Steaming. The suffocating heat under the draped towel, the red, flushed face and difficulty breathing: this is my memory of treatment for childhood colds. There's a long tradition of inhaling heated water vapor to ease congestion from colds—followed religiously by my family. But to me the cure seemed worse than the ailment. In theory, the wet heat is supposed to help thickened mucus drain away. However, a 2006 review found a mix of evidence; in some studies, steaming seemed to ease symptoms; in others it had no effect. No harm in it for adults if they're into steamy suffocation—as long as they don't burn themselves.

Stuffing or Starving. There's little evidence to support the old maxim that eating affects the course of a cold, and certainly none that avoiding food altogether shortens a cold's duration or reduces symptoms. Not long ago Dutch scientists showed that eating a meal boosts levels of gamma interferon, a natural antiviral produced by the body—but the study was tiny and has not since been replicated. However, we do know that good nutrition is essential for a healthy immune response. And whether or not eating triggers antiviral activity, it may offer comfort—a benefit not to be underestimated. Check out the recipes on pages 195–203 for some for tasty cold-comfort food offered up by experts.

Tender Loving Care (TLC) or Empathy. As Tom Ball points out, TLC from a friend or family member can go a long way in comforting cold sufferers. The same is true for empathy from a doctor. Scientists have found that a doctor's caring and compassion can reduce the duration of a cold by a full day—with no side effects.

Vicks VapoRub. This is the commercial version of those camphor rubs used by so many moms from different cultures to relieve nasal congestion in their kids. Vicks VapoRub no longer claims to be a decongestant because there's no evidence that it's effective against congestion. However, its aromatic ingredients, especially menthol, may create the sensation of coolness in the nose, which can make some stuffy noses feel more open. In general, it's considered safe when used as directed but has little or no medicinal value—and for children, it may be dangerous. In 2009, a report showed that when the rub is used on infants and toddlers just below the nose, it can cause airway inflammation and severe respiratory distress.

Vinegar Gargle. I have friends—university professors, normally very sober, skeptical types—who swear by this old folk remedy. As soon as they feel the first tickle or scratchiness in their throat, they drop everything to gargle with the vinegar, and so they claim, the cold never materializes. Because of the depth of their conviction, I scoured the literature to find confirmation or a possible mechanism of action. As far as I can tell there's little if any clinical evidence. I did discover that vinegar has a low pH—around 2.4, which is pretty acidic. Lab studies have found that rhinoviruses are inactivated by low pH, says Ron Turner, but whether this can be applied to people is highly questionable. "Our bodies are designed to not let something within us stay at a low pH for any length of time—the body quickly normalizes pH by secreting proteins," he explains. "In any case, gargling would not reach the adenoids, where rhinoviruses launch their infection. When we gargle, the soft palate closes off this area." (Otherwise, gargling would make you choke.) So, says Turner, "your friends are gargling where the rhinovirus isn't." Do I tell them this and risk ruining their placebo effect?

Vitamin C (also called ascorbic acid). There's probably no home remedy better studied than the Big C. The upshot of all the research, however, is the disappointing news that when it comes to cold prevention and therapy, C mostly gets a D. Taking the vitamin regularly does little to ward off colds—unless you're a true believer (in which case the placebo effect may kick in) or an elite athlete or a soldier in extreme conditions. In 2004, the Cochrane Collaboration reviewed all the legitimate evidence—30 studies of more than 11,000 people—and concluded that taking the vitamin on a regular basis does not help to prevent colds in the general population. It may reduce the duration and severity of symptoms but only very slightly— probably because of its anticholinergic activity, which dries up secretions, says Jack Gwaltney Jr. But Gwaltney feels that antihistamines are more effective at doing this.

There may be some benefit for people living in extreme conditions, such as soldiers, skiers, and marathon runners engaged in endurance exercise or exposed to very cold environments. Studies suggest that for these "extremists," downing a daily dose of 200 milligrams of C reduces the incidence of colds by half.

Most experts agree that taking daily vitamin C does not prevent colds or ease symptoms once you have one but may shorten cold a fraction—by about 10 percent in adults; 15 percent in children.

(Note: Normal doses of vitamin C—around 100 milligrams daily, easily obtained through a diet rich in fruits and vegetables—are generally safe in healthy people. Very large doses can result in diarrhea.)

Vitamin D. Vitamin D has become the new white hope for everything from bone health to cancer prevention. Lately, it has entered the spotlight as a nutrient that may possibly normalize the body's immune response, reducing the incidence and severity of cold symptoms. In 2009, a study looking at the vitamin D levels, nutritional habits, and rates of respiratory infection of almost 19,000 men and women found that people with low levels of vitamin D (10 nanograms per milliliter) were 40 percent more likely to have had a recent respiratory infection than those with high levels (more than 30 nanograms per milliliter). (People with asthma or chronic obstructive pulmonary disease seemed to be at special risk: low levels of D magnified manifold their apparent vulnerability to infection compared with people without lung disease.) However, epidemiological studies such as this one don't necessarily show cause and effect. To understand whether vitamin D actually prevents colds, scientists need to conduct randomized, placebo-controlled studies—where they give some people the vitamin and others placebo for a period of time—and then see who's more likely to come down with a cold.

Still, it's a good idea to have your D levels checked, and

if they're low, talk to your physician about raising them with the help of supplements. We get vitamin D naturally through diet and exposure to sunlight. Dietary sources of vitamin D include fatty fish, such as salmon, tuna, and mackerel, and to a lesser degree egg yolks and cheese. But it is nearly impossible to get sufficient amounts of the vitamin from diet alone—and not easy to keep levels optimal through sunlight exposure, especially if you live at high latitudes. Studies suggest that more than a third of adults in this country have suboptimal blood levels of vitamin D. If your blood levels are low or marginal, experts recommend taking vitamin D in supplement form, 1,000 international units per day.

Zicam. A homeopathic remedy containing minuscule amounts of zinc, Zicam is touted by its makers, Matrixx Initiatives, as "specially formulated to shorten your colds so you don't just feel better—you ARE better, sooner." There's little evidence to support the claim (see Zinc below), and now it seems there may be risk associated with some Zicam products. In 2009 the FDA advised the public to stop using Zicam nasal gel and nasal swabs because of their association with the loss of the sense of smell (anosmia). Says UVA cold researcher Ron Turner, "Can I imagine using this stuff? No way. To take something that does little good and that may cause me to lose my sense of smell is just not worth it."

Zinc. Over the past two decades or so, the use of zinc as a cure for the common cold (primarily in the form of lozenges and nasal sprays and gels) has grown in popularity. An essential mineral found throughout the body, zinc is needed for growth, wound healing, and immune function. In the lab, it has been shown to inhibit the growth of rhinoviruses, but only at near-toxic concentrations; it shows no antiviral activity against rhinovirus infections in human volunteers. The clinical studies of zinc's impact on colds have been all over the map. This is in large part because many of the studies are flawed. In 2007, a Stanford University review of 105 trials conducted over the past 20 years found only 14 that were well designed and controlled. The highest-quality trials indicated that zinc had no impact on the course of colds. In those studies that showed some benefit, zinc was most effective if taken in the form of nasal spray within 48 hours of the start of symptoms. However, the FDA advises against taking zinc directly in the nose through sprays or gels, as this may result in permanent damage to the sense of smell. More common side effects include bad taste and nausea.

Get This

A Guide to Cold-Care and Prevention Products for the Comfort-Craving, Fashion-Conscious, or High-Tech Germaphobe

Balm-y Aid for Red and Chafed Nose. I find that there's nothing better to soothe those red and irritated nostrils than a dab of Vermont's Original Bag Balm. Created more than 100 years ago to soften cow udders, Bag Balm contains petroleum and lanolin and doubles as a handy salve for nipples sore from nursing or for bike butt. It comes in the original little green can with red clover and a cow's head. ($8 at drugstores, hardware stores, farm and feed stores, pet shops, and tack shops)

Throat Relief. Most experts agree that so-called demulcents (from the Latin *demulcere*, meaning "to soothe" or "to caress") can help to relieve a sore or scratchy throat caused by the irritation of inflamed mucous membranes. Two of my favorites are Ricola herbal cough drops (about $2 for 24 drops, available at most pharmacies) and the outrageously expensive blackcurrant-flavored Grether's Pastilles, made in Switzerland from an old English formula. ($12 for 4 ounces)

Sock It to You. This has nothing to do with that cocka-mamie concept of cold-sock treatment, a "hydrotherapy" technique that involves going to bed in cold, wet socks to relieve nasal congestion at night. No, this is just a perfect pair of cozy socks—Brookstone's Nap Travel Socks, made of "ultra-plush NapSoft® material"—to keep the tootsies warm when you've got the chills and to promote that healing nap. ($10 at www.Brookstone.com)

If You Can't Outfight 'Em, Out-Fashion 'Em with an eye-catching rhinovirus necktie or bowtie ("butterfly-winged, manual tying, coup de cravat!"). The striking rhino-virus design is available in black and purple or burgundy and tan on 100 percent silk. Ties are made by Infectious Aware-ables, defined as "a rapidly emerging, non-resistant strain of AWAREness agents." The company advertises that a portion of the proceeds from its sales is donated to research or educa-tion on infectious disease. Says *People Magazine*, "The ties are spreading like swine flu." ($39.95 at www.iawareables.com)

Stylish "Sniffs." For fashionistas, designer tissues printed in a Mona Lisa design, leopard print, zebra print, camouflage, or my favorite, $100 bills. (6 "Sniff" packets for $9.95 at drug-stores, novelty shops, and online)

The Scoop on Hand Sanitizers. For beating cold bugs, nothing beats thorough hand washing with soap and water.

(Use regular soap; antibacterial soaps are no more effective against cold germs.) But if you can't wash your hands, a half-teaspoon or so of an alcohol-based hand sanitizer such as Purell or Germ-X is a decent second choice. There's not much data on whether sanitizers effectively disable viruses, but they do make your hands less hospitable to the bugs. Choose carefully: the CDC advises using products with at least a 60 percent alcohol content, preferably higher. (Available at drugstores, grocery stores, and other outlets; $2–$8 for 8 ounces.)

Killer Tissues. Antiviral tissues made by Kleenex claim to "kill" 99.9 percent of the most common kinds of cold viruses within 15 minutes of contact. This doesn't do much for the nose-blower. But theoretically it might help to prevent the spread of a virus by sparing the unsuspecting handler of used tissues. ($2 for a box of 120, available at drugstores and grocery stores)

TripStixx. For the traveler in Asia discomfited by the concept of using secondhand chopsticks, a set of personal sticks—portable, hygienic, easily washable—featuring one set of handles with two detachable tips, one for sushi, the other for Chinese banquet dishes such as stir-fried beef. (About $15 at www.tripstixx.com)

The Handler. If you're the type who longs for latex gloves as a second skin, this germ-fighting key fob is for you. Marketed as a viable alternative to using your bare hands, it's a little mechanical device with a pop-out hook that allows you to avoid touching public surfaces—door handles, elevator buttons, hotel remotes, ATM keypads, paper towel dispensers, etc. (About $11 at pharmacies and at www.handlerusa .com)

The Germ Slayer. Otherwise known as the H1N1 Destroying UV Wand from Hammacher Schlemmer. Take the hype with a big grain of salt. Using UV-C light ("the same kind trusted to sterilize hospital instruments"), this hand-held germ-killing wand claims to eradicate up to 99.9 percent of bacteria, viruses, and mold in 20 seconds. Hold the device three inches above a surface—cutting board, keyboard, telephone, baby toys, cribs, strollers—and it supposedly zaps the DNA of microorganisms that cause the flu and the common cold. (About $70 at www.hammacher.com) A cheaper version is the Pocket Purifier, which retails for about $20. But here's the boulder of salt: "There's no question that UV light kills germs," says Harley Rotbart. "And UV lights are a great technique for irradiating surfaces where scientists are working with serious strains of bubonic plague. But the bugs have to be exposed to the light long enough for it to mutate their DNA." In other words, a quick zap is unlikely to do the trick.

Germ Guardian Nursery Sanitizer. For sanitizing toys, pacifiers, bottles, and other baby items. The sanitizer uses heat rather than chemicals to kill some cold viruses and other germs. However, many consumers complain that the chamber is too small to be truly useful. ($70 at department stores and online at www.guardiantechnologies.com)

Henry the Hand's Health Shield. This clear plastic face shield is the brainchild of the Henry the Hand Foundation and Henry the Hand Champion Handwasher, a nonprofit organization devoted to making the public more aware of the role of hands in spreading disease. The shield enforces the "barrier" method of protection, preventing wearers from putting their fingers in eyes, nose, or mouth—but it's a little cumbersome to say the least. ($2 per shield, available at www.henrythehand .com)

Kleanly Keyboards. Two contraptions: The WETKEYS Washable Wireless Keyboard is a single piece of molded silicone that can be removed and washed with soap and water to eliminate germs. ($60 at www.wetkeys.com) Vioguard is developing the first self-sanitizing computer keyboard, which uses germicidal UV-C light to kill bacteria and viruses. The product is designed for use in hospitals but may find a wider market among those who obsess over contaminated keyboards. ($499 to $599 at www.vioguard.com)

Sanitary Cell Phones. In 2009, Scottish microbiologists released a study suggesting that cell phones carry more germs per square inch than just about any surface—door handle, toilet seat, sole of a shoe. One company seized on the opportunity to market Cleen Cell Wet Wipes, premoistened with a disinfectant solution that cleans germs from cell phones without harming the screen or electronics. (About $14 for 24 wipes, available at www.cleencell.com)

The Real Cure
Recipes and Readings

> I enjoy convalescence. It is the part that makes the illness worthwhile.
>
> GEORGE BERNARD SHAW

While the science of preventing or curing colds moves in marching-band fashion—a step forward, a step back, with occasional twirling in place—here are some suggestions for what is currently the only real cure for the common cold: time and the comfort of eating and reading.

There may be no validity to the old adage "Feed a cold, starve a fever," but in my book there's much to be said for eating, whether or not you're ill. When I got colds or flu as a child, my father occasionally made me a chicken soup of his mother's devising, a rich broth spiced with garlic and flecked with diced onion and parsnips. I would stay home from school, curl up in my bed, and sip Grandma's soup while I read the Narnia series or poems by Ogden Nash. No wonder I faked illness at every opportunity.

Comforting Food and Drink

Hot Toddy, Mock and Not

The popular thinking that hot drinks are good for colds has given rise to the hot toddy—by some accounts, an export from India to Great Britain.

2 tablespoons honey
1½ tablespoons fresh-squeezed lemon juice
1 cup water, brought to boil in a kettle or microwave
Optional: Add a few slices of peeled fresh ginger to the water before boiling.

Mix honey and lemon juice in a mug. Pour water over it, and stir well. To make a real hot toddy, add 1 ounce (2 tablespoons) of good bourbon, brandy, or Scotch.

Sick-on-the-Sofa Old-Fashioned

Here's a cold drink for colds, recommended by Richard Howorth, owner of Square Books in Oxford, Mississippi. "Perhaps the best thing about an old-fashioned is that if you're sick with a cold and feel well enough to have a drink, you're probably on your way to recovery," says Richard. "It's the thing my wife Lisa most wants me to make for her when she's sick, and it's the only time either of us has this particular drink. The curative aspect of an old-fashioned is that it simply helps one feel a bit better about what one is already doing—lying on the sofa, reading, watching bad TV, and falling asleep."

Fairly large glass, so as to accommodate the fruit

1½ ounces bourbon (Any brand will do, as it will be compromised by the other ingredients and, anyway, the patient's taste buds are already shot. Use more or less, depending on how you're feeling.)

Soda water

Bitters (the only time we use this in our house, I believe)

1 scant teaspoon sugar

Ice, of course (crushed, if the bartender is up to it, but certainly not necessary)

Citrus fruit (a couple of sections of grapefruit, several sections of orange, or half a clementine—or you can use smaller quantities of all these in combination)

Maraschino cherry (we keep a small jar in the fridge; also the only time we use these)

Pour bourbon into glass. Add a splash of soda water, a dash of bitters, and sugar. Stir with a spoon to dissolve the sugar. Then add ice. Cut, peel, and add a generous slice of fruit. Add some soda water. Stir just a bit more to get the fruit on the bottom and to chill the drink. Add a lemon twist if you want to get fancy. Put a cherry on top (necessary). Sip and eat the fruit in the order you prefer (using fingers)—but the cherry, following the sugary dregs of this drink, should go last. Soon you will be well.

(Note of caution: Though a hot toddy or an old-fashioned can take the sting out of cold misery, too much alcohol may cause dehydration, prolonging symptoms.)

Banana Pudding

This version of the southern classic lacks the decadence of vanilla wafers and whipped cream, which you can add at the end if you like.

1 cup sugar
¼ cup cornstarch or ½ cup flour
¼ teaspoon salt
4 egg yolks
2 cups whole milk
1 tablespoon unsalted butter, cut into pieces
1 teaspoon vanilla extract
A couple of ripe bananas, peeled and sliced

Mix together the sugar, cornstarch or flour, and salt in a bowl. In a small bowl, beat the egg yolks well, then pour into heavy saucepan and place over medium heat. To the egg yolks, add the sugar/flour mixture, alternating with the milk, whisking constantly. When the mixture starts to bubble, reduce heat to low, and continue to whisk until mixture begins to thicken, another minute or two. Add butter and vanilla, and continue to stir to prevent scorching. When the mixture reaches pudding consistency, remove from heat. Place plastic wrap on surface of pudding to prevent the formation of skin. Chill for at least a few hours. Whisk again before serving, then fold in sliced bananas.

Buttermilk Biscuits

These biscuits are delicious—crisp on the outside, tender and airy in the middle—perfect vehicles for a healing smear of strawberry preserves or honey.

2 cups flour
½ teaspoon baking soda
2 teaspoons baking powder
¾ teaspoon salt
½ teaspoon sugar
½ cup (1 stick) unsalted butter, cut into pieces (plus 2 tablespoons
for brushing on top of biscuits)
1 cup buttermilk

Preheat the oven to 375 degrees Fahrenheit. Mix together all dry ingredients in a bowl. Cut in butter until mixture resembles coarse crumbs. (You can also do this with the help of a food processor: Put half the mixture into the processor along with the butter, and pulse until the biggest pieces are pea size. Then add this to the remaining flour mixture, and pinch with fingers to combine.) Blend in enough buttermilk so the mixture comes together and the dough leaves the sides of the bowl. It will be sticky. On a lightly floured surface, turn the dough out and pat it into a thickness of 1 inch or so. Cut with a large, round biscuit cutter. Line a baking sheet with parchment paper, and put biscuits on sheet. Bake until golden brown, around 18 minutes. Cool for a few minutes on a wire rack.

Chicken Soups for the Cold Soul

Because of the hen's alleged healing powers, I offer two recipes for chicken soup, one belonging to Barbara Rennard, wife of Dr. Stephen Rennard, who conducted the first research on the soup's possible medicinal effects on the common cold, and one conceived by Lynne Rossetto Kasper, cookbook author and host of *The Splendid Table*.

Grandma's Chicken Soup Recipe
by Barbara Rennard

A decade ago, Stephen Rennard, professor of medicine at the University of Nebraska Medical Center, published the first study showing that chicken soup may have some anti-inflammatory benefits. His curiosity about the healing effects of chicken soup arose from his wife's conviction that her Lithuanian grandmother's chicken soup was effective in treating colds in their family. Here's the recipe.

One 5- to 6-pound stewing hen or baking chicken
One 2- to 4-pound package of chicken wings
3 large onions
1 large sweet potato
3 parsnips
2 turnips
11 to 12 large carrots
5 to 6 celery stems
1 bunch of parsley
Salt and pepper, to taste

Clean the chicken. Put it in a large pot, and cover it with cold water. Bring the water to boil. Peel the root vegetables. Add the chicken wings, onions, sweet potato, parsnips, turnips, and carrots. Boil about 1½ hours. Remove fat from the surface as it accumulates. Add the celery and parsley. Cook the mixture about 45 minutes longer. Remove the chicken. The chicken is not used further for the soup. (The meat makes excellent chicken parmesan.) Put the vegetables in a food processor until they are chopped fine, or pass them through a strainer. Add salt and pepper to taste. (Note: This soup freezes well.)

Brodo di Mamma, or Mother's Broth,
by Lynne Rossetto Kasper

(*from* The Italian Country Table: Home Cooking from Italy's Farmhouse Kitchens *by Lynne Rossetto Kasper, Scribner, 1999*)

Chef Lynne Rossetto Kasper is one of my heroes, author of three exquisite cookbooks, and host of a public radio program on food and cooking, *The Splendid Table*. Whenever I'm in need of sumptuous comfort food, I turn to her cookbook, *The Splendid Table's How to Eat Supper*. When I asked Lynne for her favorite food to comfort the ailing, she sent me her recipe for Brodo di Mamma (including an adaptation of "The Cure" for children), along with these notes:

The mother in this broth's title is mine. For years, I'd been gathering broth-making advice from Italian friends, but it didn't all come together until my mother had major surgery. She's Italian and loves to eat. So when she lost all interest in food, we got worried. So did her doctor. She had to eat, he said, an instruction that could throw the Italian army into action. "Make broth" was all I could think. It was like winnowing everything I'd ever learned about stock making. I used only organic ingredients. I simmered the broth a long time to draw out every nutrient and seasoned it with tomatoes and great heads of garlic instead of the salt my mother could no longer use. I made buckets of it, and she ate every bit. Her surgery was six years ago. Mom is now 89 and gives dinner parties on a regular basis. We still make the broth. With its track record, why take chances?

Whole heads of garlic, juicy tomatoes, and overnight simmering are what give this poultry broth its extraordinarily deep and full flavors. Valentino Marcattili of Ristorante San Domenico in Imola first told me about using turkey wings for broth instead of Italy's more traditional capon. Since wings are neither dark meat nor white, but somewhere in between, the broth they give is substantial yet subtle. Putting a few tomatoes in the pot is an old Italian trick for giving the liquid its appealing edge. Garlic deepens and enriches, yet leaves no detectable garlicky taste. Long cooking coaxes every bit of flavor and nutrition from the ingredients, an economy honored by so many country cooks.

This is the broth you make to cook the wonderful tortellini from your favorite pasta shop. This is the broth you make for your own homemade pasta. This is the broth you make for your daughter's wedding soup or for your own birthday. This broth could even seduce a hesitant lover into commitment.

And it keeps in the freezer for months—up to six, in fact.

Cook to cook: If possible, use organic vegetables and poultry raised on organic feed without antibiotics and drugs. Freeze some of the broth in ice cube trays (turning out cubes into plastic bags once they are frozen). Each cube equals about 2 tablespoons. Freeze the remainder of the broth in assorted-sized containers for up to 6 months.

Makes about 7 quarts.

5 pounds turkey wings or 5 pounds whole chicken (if possible, hormone- and antibiotic-free)
About 6 quarts cold water
2 large onions (1½ pounds), trimmed of root ends and coarsely chopped (do not peel)

2 medium carrots, coarsely chopped
1 large stalk celery with leaves, coarsely chopped
4 large heads garlic, trimmed of root ends and halved horizontally
2 whole cloves garlic
1 bay leaf, broken
6 canned tomatoes, drained

Cut up the turkey wings or chicken, cracking the bones with a cleaver in two or three places. Place in an 8- to 10-quart stockpot. Add enough cold water to come to within 3 inches of the lip of the pot. Bring the water slowly to a simmer. Skim off all the foam. Add the remaining ingredients, partially cover the pot, and bring to a slow bubble. Simmer 12 to 14 hours, occasionally stirring and skimming off fat. Do not boil the broth. Keep the liquid bubbling very slowly. Add boiling water if the broth reduces below the level of the solid ingredients; always keep them covered with about 3 inches of liquid.

Strain the broth through a fine sieve. For a clearer broth, strain it by ladling rather than pouring, leaving behind any sediment at the bottom of the pot. Cool the broth as quickly as possible. Set it outside in cold weather, or chill it in several small containers set in bowls of ice. Then refrigerate the broth for about 8 hours, or until its fat has hardened. Skim off the hardened fat, and freeze in assorted-sized containers.

Making Simple Soups with Mother's Broth

    "The Cure": Every child in Italy has known the
        nourishment of a bowl of tiny pasta cooked
        in homemade broth and finished with grated
        Parmigiano-Reggiano cheese. It made being sick in
        bed almost worthwhile. Use any small shape that
        pleases you.

Brodo con Prosciutto: A dinner-party soup of seasoned broth brought to a boil, ladled into bowls, and garnished with thin strips of prosciutto di Parma. A few leaves of parsley finish the dish.

Summer Broth with Herbs: Simmer broth, and season to taste. Stir into each serving a tablespoon of mixed fresh herbs, coarsely chopped. Pass grated Parmigiano-Reggiano at the table.

Apristomaco (Tummy Opener): An old and playful word, meaning a light teaser for awakening appetites. In this case a few thin slices of soaked dried porcini mushrooms, slivers of scallion, and basil leaves are floated in hot, seasoned broth.

Readings

The cold should not be treated with contempt, but followed by bed rest, a good book to read...

SIR WILLIAM OSLER

What books warm the bones when you're down with a cold? Here's a smattering of suggestions from experts around the country.

Cold Classics: Roxanne Coady of R. J. Julia Booksellers in Madison, Connecticut, recommends Anthony Trollope's six novels about wealthy aristocrat and politician Plantagenet Palliser and his wife, Lady Glencora. Rachael Amos of the Tattered Cover Book Store in Denver, Colorado, votes for *Pride and Prejudice* "because it's so familiar it's like having someone tell you a story while you're lying there, and it's so good that you always notice something you hadn't noticed before." Roberta Rubin, the owner of the Book Stall at Chestnut Court in Winnetka, Illinois, recommends Jane Austen, Charles Dickens, and Edith Wharton.

Alice in Wonderland is the choice of Cathy Langer (also from the Tattered Cover). "When I was sick as a child, my mother would set me up for the day in her double bed, portable record player next to me, with the unabridged *Alice in Wonderland* on records. It turned a day at home with a cold into a special treat."

Escapism, another common cold genre: Emilio Esquibel, a bookseller at the Tattered Cover, was in bed for a year when he was 12, recovering from rheumatic fever, so he is an expert on escapist literature. He recommends anything by Lee Child; and for men, Daniel Silva's series about a spy and assassin for the Israeli secret service. Roxanne Coady suggests Harlan Coben's books. Cathy Langer likes to recommend the series that got her through a bad bout of West Nile virus: Alexander McCall Smith's No. 1 Ladies' Detective Agency series. ("Light and engaging," says Langer, "they take you far away to dry and sunny Botswana where Precious Ramotswe is the eminently sensible and cunning proprietor of a detective agency.") Smith is Roberta Rubin's choice, too, along with a few other mystery writers (Donna Leon, Deborah Crombie, and Robert Parker), as well as "not-too-heavy novels to prop up in bed," such as *The Guernsey Literary and Potato Peel Pie Society* by Mary Ann Shaffer, *The Girl Who Played with Fire* by Stieg Larsson, and Garth Stein's *The Art of Racing in the Rain.*

For the Out-of-Humor: Laughter heals. Cathy Langer recommends the *New Yorker* humor compilations *Fierce Pajamas* and *Disquiet Please.* "Anthologies are great for dipping into between naps," she says. "You don't have to remember where you were, follow a plot, or keep track of characters." For wit and charm, Roxanne Coady recommends James Thurber and E. B. White's *Is Sex Necessary?* and Elaine Dundy, *The Dud Avocado.* To humor the hypochondriac, Susannah Vazehgoo of Porter Square Books in Boston heartily recommends an old favorite: *Three Men in a*

Boat (To Say Nothing of the Dog) by Jerome K. Jerome, originally published in 1889. "The book starts off with the narrator reading a medical dictionary, and by the time he is done he is certain he has every ailment known to man," she writes. "In order to forget his medical woes and to best spend his last days on earth enjoying himself, he plans a vacation with his two best chums (and a dog), rowing a boat down the Thames and camping on its banks each night. The book is a little gem," she says, "very humorous, in a droll, clever kind of way, just the kind of book to distract you from your stuffy nose and aching sinuses!"

And finally, for the nasal gazers among us…a few notable cold quotations and anecdotes:

"To be sick is to enjoy monarchical prerogatives."
CHARLES LAMB

"The first rule laid down for preventing colds, is to harden the body, by enuring it daily to bear the open air."
WILLIAM BUCHAN, *Domestic Medicine* (1769)

Writer Robert Benchley's anticold regimen: "Don't breathe through your nose or mouth."

"The Best Preventive of Colds is to wash your children every day thoroughly in cold water, if they are strong enough to bear it; if not, add a little warm water, and rub the skin dry."
SARAH JOSEPHA HALE, *The Good Housekeeper* (1839)

"My own remedy is always to eat, just before I step into bed, a hot roasted onion."
GEORGE WASHINGTON (ATTRIBUTED)

"A disagreeable tickling in the throat, causing a
constant provocation to cough, is sometimes so
importunate as to force the patient to have recourse to
various means of procuring some present relief: a few
raisins will sometimes answer this purpose."

WILLIAM HEBERDEN, *Commentaries on the
History and Cure of Diseases* (1798)

"I feel rather languid and solitary—perhaps because I
have a cold..."

JANE AUSTEN, in a letter to her sister Cassandra
(June 15, 1808)

Austen, who speaks often of colds in her letters, was fond
of penalizing her heroines with wicked colds for their careless
disregard of poor weather. In *Sense and Sensibility*, poor Mari-
anne Dashwood's walk through the wet grass at twilight and
sitting afterward in "wet shoes and stockings" nearly results
in her death from

a cold so violent, as, though for a day or two trifled with
or denied, would force itself by increasing ailments, on
the concern of every body, and the notice of herself. Prescriptions poured in from all quarters, and as usual,
were all declined. Though heavy and feverish, with a
pain in her limbs, a cough, and a sore throat, a good
night's rest was to cure her entirely; and it was with difficulty that Elinor prevailed on her, when she went to
bed, to try one or two of the simplest of the remedies.

In an age when most people were lucky to live to 60, Jane
Austen's contemporary, Thomas Jefferson, made it to the age
of 83 and only very rarely suffered a cold. His secret? Soaking

his feet in cold water—or so he claimed. This despite his dread of feeling cold: "I have no doubt but that cold is the source of more suffering to all animal nature than hunger, thirst, sickness, and all other pains of life and of death itself put together," he wrote in 1801. And yet, every morning, from the time he was a young man in Williamsburg until his death, Jefferson soaked his feet in a bucket of icy water. "I am fortunate in health," he opined at the age of 76, "so free from catarrhs that I have not had one on an average of eight or ten years through life. I ascribe this exemption partly to the habit of bathing my feet in cold water every morning, for sixty years past."

Charles Lamb, poet, essayist, and critic of the late 18th and early 19th centuries, was a fine correspondent; his letters include this singular complaint of a severe cold, addressed to his friend, Quaker poet Bernard Barton, on January 9, 1824 (from which I've cannibalized several lines for use in this book):

Dear B.B.,—Do you know what it is to succumb under an insurmountable day-mare,—"a whoreson lethargy," Falstaff calls it,—an indisposition to do anything or to be anything; a total deadness and distaste; a suspension of vitality; an indifference to locality; a numb, soporific good-for-nothingness; an ossification all over; an oyster-like insensibility to the passing events; a mind-stupor; a brawny defiance to the needles of a thrusting-in conscience? Did you ever have a very bad cold, with a total irresolution to submit to water-gruel processes? This has been for many weeks my lot and my excuse. My fingers drag heavily over this paper, and to my thinking it is three-and-twenty furlongs from here to the end of this demi-sheet. I have not a thing to say; nothing is of more importance than another. I am flatter than a denial or a pancake; emptier than Judge Parke's wig when the head is in it; duller than a country stage when the actors are off it,—a cipher, an o! I acknowledge life at all only by an occasional convulsional cough and a permanent phlegmatic pain in the chest. I am weary of the world; life is weary of me. My day is gone into twilight, and I don't think it worth the expense of candles. My wick hath a thief in it, but I can't muster courage to snuff it. I inhale suffocation; I can't distinguish veal from mutton; nothing interests me. 'Tis twelve o'clock, and Thurtell is just now coming out upon the new drop, Jack Ketch alertly tucking up his greasy sleeves to do the last office of mortality; yet cannot I elicit a groan or a moral reflection. If you told me the world will be at an end to-morrow, I should just say, "Will it?" I have not volition enough left to dot my i's, much less to comb my eyebrows; my eyes are set in my head; my brains are gone out to see a poor relation in Moorfields, and they did not say when they'd come back again; my skull is a Grub Street attic to let,—not so much as a joint-stool left in it; my hand writes, not I, from habit, as chickens run about a little when their heads are off. Oh for a vigorous fit of gout, colic, toothache,—an earwig in my auditory, a fly in my visual organs; pain is life,—the sharper the more evidence of life; but this apathy, this death! Did you ever have an obstinate cold,—a six or seven weeks' unintermitting chill and suspension of hope, fear, conscience, and everything? Yet do I try all I can to cure it. I try wine, and spirits, and smoking, and snuff in unsparing quantities; but they all only seem to make me worse, instead of better. I sleep in a damp room, but it does me no good; I come home late o' nights, but do not find any visible amendment! Who shall deliver me from the body of this death?

ACKNOWLEDGMENTS

My muse for this book was my friend and fellow writer Mark Edmundson, who has suffered his share of tigerlike colds over the years, and who suggested that the world needed a little book on the topic and even offered up a catchy title. Profound thanks, Mark, and may the remainder of your days be sniffle-free.

I would like to express my deepest appreciation to the scientists and researchers at the University of Virginia (UVA) who have devoted their careers to the study of the common cold and who freely and generously shared their expertise with me: Jack Gwaltney Jr., Birgit Winther, Ron Turner, and Owen Hendley. This book would not have been possible without them. I would also like to thank Annie Tromey and Betty Lang, nurses in the UVA cold study program, for relating tales of previous cold studies and for their superb competence, humor, and good cheer.

Several scientists took considerable time and care in explaining their research to me. I am grateful to Thomas Ball of the University of Arizona Health Sciences Center, Sheldon Cohen of Carnegie Mellon University, Yori Gidron of Brunel University, Sebastian Johnston of Imperial College London, Elaine Larson of Columbia University, Harley Rotbart of the Children's Hospital of Denver, and Jacqueline Shan of Afexa Life Sciences and the University of Alberta. For their helpful email correspondence, I'd like to thank Bruce Barrett of the University of Wisconsin, Bernhard Baune of James Cook University, Romola Bucks of the University of Western Australia, Christopher Drake of the Henry Ford Hospital Sleep Center, Giovanni Fontana of the Università degli studi di Firenze, Charles

Gerba of the University of Arizona, and Sunita Vohra of the University of Alberta.

I'm extremely grateful to Angela Greenslade and Janet Wilson-Ward for our delightful time together in London and for sharing their stories about their "holidays" at the Common Cold Unit. I found Angela through her blog post about the CCU; that she responded to my query with such open generosity touched me. Heartfelt thanks also to my dear friend Cathy (who prefers to remain anonymous) for relating her germaphobic view of the world.

In addition, I appreciate the communications of Warren Michaels of Afexa Life Sciences about COLD-FX and the help of Judy Budreau of American Public Media.

For supplying sublimely delicious cold-comfort recipes, I am indebted to my old friend Richard Howorth, owner of Square Books and mayor of Oxford, Mississippi; Lynne Rossetto Kasper, luminous host of *The Splendid Table* and author of several bestselling cookbooks; and Barbara and Stephen Rennard (chief of pulmonary medicine at the University of Nebraska Medical Center) of Omaha, Nebraska.

When I solicited booksellers for ideas about especially entertaining sick-bed reading, a number responded generously with excellent suggestions. Many thanks to Rachael Amos, Emilio Esquibel, and Cathy Langer of the Tattered Cover Book Store in Denver; Susannah Vazehgoo and Ellen Jarrett of Porter Square Books in Boston; Roxanne J. Coady of R. J. Julia Booksellers in Madison, Connecticut; and Roberta Rubin of the Book Stall at Chestnut Park in Winnetka, Illinois.

I am hugely grateful to Melanie Jackson, my incomparable agent, for landing this book in the hands of the ingenious and creative Jonathan Karp. Thank you, Melanie, for your warm support over the years and for finding the perfect editor for this book; and thank you, Jon, for your faith in the book, your inspiring editorial insights, and your stoicism in staying at the job despite round-the-calendar colds. I also appreciate the capable, energetic assistance of the staff at Twelve, including Cary Goldstein and Colin Shepherd.

I would like to thank my friends who supported me in innumerable ways through the writing of this book, most especially filmmaker Paul Wagner, who created the excellent little video for *Ah-Choo!* and Mim Nelson and Kin Earle, who read the manuscript in draft form and buoyed my spirits from afar.

Finally, I could never find words to adequately thank my two daughters, Zoë and Nell, and my husband, Karl, for the myriad ways they nurture me and make my writing possible; they are the three who make me one.

NOTES

Introduction: The Cold Truth

The description of Wally Schirra's spaceflight is drawn from the Wally Schirra memorial website: www.wallyschirra.com and http://history.nasa .gov/SP-368/s2ch1.htm.

Calculations of suffering caused by the common cold come from S. Kirchberger, "Modulation of the immune system by human rhinoviruses," *Int Arch Allergy Immunol* 142: 1–10 (2007). The cartoon about the job of a cold researcher can be found in Tyrrell and Fielder (2002), p. 60. Harley Rotbart's quotation occurs in Rotbart (2008), p. 43. The economic costs of the common cold are quantified in A. Mark Fendrick et al., "The economic burden of non-influenza-related viral respiratory tract infection in the United States," *Arch Intern Med* 163: 487–94 (2003); and Gregory A. Poland and Michael A. Barry, "Common cold, uncommon variation," *New Engl J Med* 360: 21 (2009). The data on absenteeism comes from P. F. Adams et al., "Current estimates from the National Health Interview Survey," *Vital Health Statistics* 10, No. 200: 59, 66 (1999).

Chapter 1: In Cold Pursuit

Birgit Winther's study on the travel of cold viruses down the lacrimal duct can be found in B. Winther et al., "Sites of rhinovirus recovery after point inoculation of the upper airway, *J Am Med Assoc* 256: 1763–7 (1986). Full descriptions of the origin of cold symptoms and the body's response to the presence of cold viruses occur in Eccles (2007); Kirchberger (2007);

J. M. Gwaltney et al., "Symptom severity patterns in experimental common colds and their usefulness in timing onset of illness in natural colds," *Clin Infect Dis* 36: 714–23 (2003); D. E. Pappas et al., "Symptom profile of common colds in school-aged children," *Ped Infect Dis* 27 (1): 8–11 (2008); and at the website www.commoncold.org. See also D. F. Proctor and I. B. Andersen, *The Nose* (Amsterdam: Elsevier Biomedical Press, 1982), pp. 203–4; R. Eccles, "A role for the nasal cycle in respiratory defence," *Eur Respir J* 9: 371–6 (1996); and J. M. Gwaltney et al., "Nose blowing propels nasal fluid into the paranasal sinuses," *Clin Infect Dis* 30: 387–91 (2000). Descriptions of the physiology of coughing can be found in J. G. Widdicombe, "Neurophysiology of the cough reflex," *Eur Respir J* 8: 1193–1202 (1995); and M. R. Pratter, "Cough and the common cold," *Chest* 129: 72S–74S (2006). The study linking Sue's demise with sore throat is E. D. S. Wolff et al., "Common avian infection plagued the tyrant dinosaurs," *PLoS ONE* 4 (9): e7288 (2009). The effect of swearing on pain can be found in Richard Stephens et al., "Swearing as a response to pain," *NeuroReport* 20 (12): 1056–60 (2009).

Chapter 2: It's Catching

Information on cold transmission can be found in J. O. Hendley and J. M. Gwaltney, "Mechanisms of transmission of rhinovirus infections," *Epidemiol Rev* 10: 242–58 (1988); and J. M. Samet, "How do we catch colds?" *Am J Resp Crit Care Med* 169: 1175–6 (2004).

Sir Christopher Andrewes describes his research on cold transmission and his work at the Common Cold Unit in Salisbury, England, in Andrewes (1973); and C. H. Andrewes, "Adventures among viruses III: The puzzle of the common cold," *New Engl J Med* 242: 235–40 (1950). Andrewes's Eilean nan Ron experiment can be found in C. H. Andrewes, "The complex epidemiology of respiratory virus infections, *Science* 146: 1274–7 (1964), and C. H. Andrewes, "Rhinoviruses and common colds," *Ann Rev Med* 17: 361–70 (1966). Jack Gwaltney Jr.'s State Farm Insurance study occurs in J. M. Gwaltney et al., "Rhinovirus infections in an industrial population I. The occurrence of illness," *New Engl J Med* 275: 1261–8 (1966) and J. M. Gwaltney (2002), p. 229. Dick's research occurs in D. J. D'Alessio et al., "Short-duration exposure and the transmission of rhinoviral colds," *J Infect Dis* 150 (2): 189–93 (1984) and D. J. D'Alessio et al., "Transmission of experimental rhinovirus colds in volunteer married couples," *J Infect Dis* 133 (1): 28–36 (1976). As for Eskimo kisses, Dick noted that during kissing the "lateral margins of donor and recipient noses may also touch," but this rarely results in infection.

James Lovelock's experience researching in the Common Cold Unit is discussed in Lovelock (2000) and in Andrewes (1973). The quotation from the hygiene textbook occurs in Florence Lyndon Meredith, *Hygiene* (Philadelphia, 1926), p. 414. Droplet propulsion during coughs and sneezes is discussed in F. E. Buckland and D. A. Tyrrell, "Spread of colds," *Br Med J* October 20, 1973, p. 123, and in Boone and Gerba (2007), p. 1690. Lovelock calls the handkerchief "a potent aid for organisms wishing to find a new host" in Lovelock (2000), p. 86.

The discussion of viruses on fomites and environmental surfaces is drawn from Boone and Gerba (2007); and B. L. England, "Detection of viruses on fomites," pp. 179–229 in C. P. Gerba and S. M. Goyal, ed., *Methods in Environmental Virology* (New York City: Marcel Dekker, 1982). A classic case of fomite-transmitted disease occurred in a hotel in York, England, in which half of the guests at a wedding reception suffered an attack of norovirus-induced gastroenteritis after a kitchen assistant vomited in a sink that was used the next morning to prepare potato salad. See J. Barker et al., "Spread and prevention of some common viral infections in community facilities and domestic homes," *J Appl Microbiol* 91: 7–21 (2001).

For the work of Gwaltney and Hendley on the role of hands in cold transmission, see J. M. Gwaltney (2002) and J. M. Gwaltney et al., "Hand-to-hand transmission of rhinovirus colds," *Ann Intern Med* 88: 463–7 (1973). The survey on Americans' nose-wiping habits was conducted on a sample of 1,037 Americans by the Opinion Research Corporation in September 2009 and reported in "Germ-spreading behaviors remain the norm, despite flu season concerns," posted on www.infectioncontroltoday.com, October 12, 2009. Mark Cooper's choice to avoid handshakes was reported in a *USA Today* article on December 10, 2004: "Politician won't shake hands."

Mark Nicas's study can be found in M. Nicas and D. Best, "A study quantifying the hand-to-face contact rate and its potential application to predicting respiratory tract infection," *J Occup and Environ Hyg* 5: 347–52 (2008). Hendley and Gwaltney's work on self-inoculation occurs in J. O. Hendley et al., "Transmission of rhinovirus colds by self-inoculation," *New Engl J Med* 288: 1361–4 (1973). The investigation of nose picking in schoolchildren is described in C. Andrade and B. S. Srihari, "A preliminary survey of rhinotillexomania in an adolescent sample," *J Clin Psychiatry* Jun 62 (6): 426–31 (2001).

NOTES

Elliot Dick's studies on airborne transmission of rhinovirus occur in E. C. Dick et al., "Aerosol transmission of rhinovirus colds," *J Infect Dis* 156 (3): 442–8 (1987); D. J. D'Alessio et al., "Short-duration exposure and the transmission of rhinoviral colds," *J Infect Dis* 150: 189–94 (1984). Dick's work on the disappearance of rhinovirus along a fomite chain can be found in L. C. Jennings et al., "Near disappearance of rhinovirus along a fomite transmission chain," *J Infect Dis* 158 (4): 888–92 (1988).

The study of the presence of rhinovirus in saliva and cough secretions appears in J. O. Hendley et al., "Transmission of rhinovirus colds by self-inoculation," *New Engl J Med* 288: 1361 (1973).

Gwaltney's iodine study occurs in J. M. Gwaltney et al., "Rhinovirus transmission: One if by air, two if by hand," *Am J Epidemiol* 107: 357–61 (1978). The research on coffee cup handles and other fomites is described in J. M. Gwaltney and J. O. Hendley, "Transmission of experimental rhinovirus infection by contaminated surfaces," *Am J Epidemiol* 116: 828–33 (1982). The study on the transmission of viruses using bacteriophage as a model occurs in F. Rheinbaben et al., "Transmission of viruses via contact in a household setting: Experiments using bacteriophage X174 as a model virus," *Journal of Hospital Infection* 46: 61–6 (2000).

The Australian study of virus-laden aerosols appears in K. N. Huynh et al., "A new method for sampling and detection of exhaled respiratory virus aerosols," *Clin Infect Dis* 46: 93–5 (2008).

Gerba's work on germs and public surfaces appears in K. A. Reynolds et al., "Occurrence of bacteria and biochemical markers on public surfaces. *Int J Environ Health Res* 15 (3): 225–34 (2005). The study on viruses in pediatricians' offices was presented by Diane Pappas at a poster, "Evidence of lingering germs on toys in pediatric waiting rooms," at the ICAAC/IDSA meeting in Washington, D.C., on October 18, 2008. The study of pathogens at military fitness centers in Hawaii occurs in K. A. Goldhammer, "Prospective study of bacterial and viral contamination of exercise equipment," *Clin J Sport Med* 16 (1): 34–8 (2006). The Swiss investigation of dollar bills can be found in Y. Thomas, "Survival of influenza virus on banknotes," *Appl Environ Microb* 74 (10): 3002–7 (2008).

For research on cold transmission in office settings, see J. J. Jaakola et al., "Shared office space and risk of the common cold," *Europ J Epidem* 11 (2): 213–6 (1995). For the work on respiratory viruses and ventilation in office buildings, see T. A. Myatt, "Detection of airborne rhinovirus and its relation to outdoor air supply in office environments," *Am J Respir Crit Care*

Med 169: 1187-90 (2004). Gerba's study on the presence of bacterial pathogens in the workplace is described in a press release by the Clorox Company, dated February 14, 2007 (available at www.clorox.com/pdf/germs _working_study.pdf); and one by the University of Arizona dated February 15, 2006, downloaded at http://ag.arizona.edu/media/archives/6.14.html.

Gerba's work on pathogens in the classroom can be found in K. R. Bright et al., "Occurrence of bacteria and viruses on elementary classroom surfaces and the potential role of classroom hygiene in the spread of infectious diseases," *J School Nursing* 26: 33 (2009). The study using the mosaic virus to trace transmission in child-care facilities occurs in Xi Jiang et al., "Pathogen transmission in child care settings," *J Infect Dis* 177: 881-88 (1998). Gerba's investigation of virus on surfaces in households and day-care centers appears in S. A. Boone and C. P. Gerba, "The occurrence of influenza A virus on household and day care center fomites," *J Infection* 51: 103-9 (2005).

The statistic on the doubling of cold rates for adults with infants or children in a household occurs in MacKay (2008), p. 304. For a discussion of cold transmission in the home, see D. A. Goldmann, "Transmission of viral respiratory infections in the home," *Pediatr Infect Dis J* 19 (10suppl): S97-102 (2000) and C. P. Gerba, "Application of quantitative risk assessment for formulating hygiene policy in the domestic setting," *J Infection* 43: 92-8 (2001). Gerba's studies on pathogens in the home appear in P. Rusin and C. Gerba, "Reduction of faecal coliform, coliform and heterotrophic plate count bacteria in the household kitchen and bathroom by disinfection with hypochlorite cleaners," *J Appl Microbiol* 85 (5): 819-28 (1998) and in Gerba (2001). Gerba's quotations on laundry appear in Gerba (2001), p. 97. Birgit Winther's investigation of viruses in the home was presented in a poster on "Contamination of surfaces in homes of adults with natural rhinovirus colds and transfer to fingertips during normal daily activities," at the ICAAC/IDSA meeting in Washington, D.C., on October 18, 2008.

Winther's hotel study appears in B. Winther et al., "Environmental contamination with rhinovirus and transfer to fingers of healthy individuals by daily life activity," *J Med Virol* 79 (10): 1606-10 (2007). Hendley is quoted in a press release about the study from the University of Virginia Health System dated September 29, 2006.

The University of California study on colds on jet flights occurs in J. N. Zitter et al., "Aircraft cabin air recirculation and symptoms of the common cold," *J Am Med Assoc* 288 (4): 483-6 (2002). See also K. Leder and

D. Newman, "Respiratory infections during air travel," *Int Med Journal* 35: 50–5 (2005) and M. B. Hocking, "Common cold transmission in commercial aircraft: Industry and passenger implications," *J Env Health Res* 3 (1): 7–12 (2004).

Chapter 3: The Bugs

Size comparisons with the rhinovirus are drawn from Tyrrell (2002), p. 109. Benjamin Franklin's musings on the common cold occur in a letter to Benjamin Rush, July 14, 1773. A fine history of common cold research can be found in Tyrrell (2002). See also A. Spickard, "The common cold: Past, present, and future research," *Chest* 48 (5): 545–9 (1965) and P. H. Long, "Etiology of acute upper respiratory infection (common cold)," *J Exp Med* 53: 447–70 (1931). The quotation from George Gee Jackson comes from G. G. Jackson, "Understanding of viral respiratory illnesses provided by experiments in volunteers," *Bacteriol Rev* 28 (4): 423–30 (1964), p. 423. Dochez's observations occur in A. R. Dochez, "Studies in the common cold: IV. Experimental transmission of common cold to Anthropoid apes and human beings by means of a filtrable agent," *J Exp Med* 52: 701 (1930).

My account of the life and research of the Common Cold Unit is drawn from Tyrrell (2002); D. J. Tyrrell, "The common cold—my favorite infection," *J Gen Vir* 68: 2053–61 (1987); Andrewes (1973); and interviews with Angela Greenslade and Janet Wilson-Ward. Information on Porton Down can be found at the U.K. Ministry of Defence website: www.mod.uk/DefenceInternet. Reports on the Porton Down tests and nerve gas research can be found at the BBC News website, http://news.bbc.co.uk.

Tyrrell's comment on the cells of the human nose occurs on Tyrrell (2002), p. 72.

Information on the race to identify the rhinovirus can be found in Gwaltney (2002); J. M. Gwaltney and W. S. Jordan, "Rhinovirus and respiratory disease," *Bacteriol Rev* 28 (4): 409–22 (1964); W. Pelon, "A cytopathogenic agent isolated from naval recruits with mild respiratory illness," *Proc Soc Exp Biol and Med* 94: 262–7 (1957); and W. H. Price, "The isolation of a new virus associated with respiratory clinical disease in humans," *Proc Natl Acad Sci* 42 (12): 892–96 (1956). My account of Price's discovery is drawn from Donald G. Cooley, "Visit to a common cold laboratory," *New York Times,* November 3, 1957; and "Medicine: Cold war breakthrough," *Time,* Sept. 30, 1957.

For discussion of the new discoveries of numerous strains of rhinoviruses, see K. E. Arden and I. M. MacKay, "Human rhinoviruses: coming in from the cold," *Genome Medicine* 1: 44 (2009); and A. Kistler, "Pan-viral screening of respiratory tract infections in adults with and without asthma reveals unexpected human coronavirus and human rhinovirus diversity," *J Infect Dis* 196 (6): 817-25 (2007). The University of Wisconsin study on unknown strains of rhinovirus detected in sick infants can be found in W. M. Lee et al., "A diverse group of previously unrecognized human rhinoviruses are common causes of respiratory illness in infants," *PloS ONE* 2 (10): e966 (2007). Research on the multiple strains of rhinovirus circulating within a family occurs in V. Peltola, "Rhinovirus transmission within families with children," *J Infect Dis* 197 (3): 382-9 (2008). The report on the genomic sequencing of rhinoviruses can be found in C. Tapparel et al., "New complete genome sequences of human rhinoviruses shed light on their phylogeny and genomic features," *BioMedCentral Genomics* 8: 224 (2007).

Seasonality of cold viruses is addressed in J. M. Gwaltney and in R. Eccles, "An explanation for the seasonality of acute upper respiratory tract viral infections," *Acta Otolaryngol* 122: 183-91 (2002). The study on the evolution of human metapneumovirus appears in M. de Graaf et al., "Evolutionary dynamics of human and avian metapneumoviruses," *J Gen Virol* 89 (Pt 12): 2933-42 (2008). Information on the possible role of adenoviruses in obesity can be found in R. L. Atkinson, "Viruses as an etiology of obesity," *Mayo Clin Proc* 82 (10): 1192-8 (2007). The characterization of the "borrowed life" of viruses comes from virologists Marc H. V. van Regenmortel of the University of Strasbourg in France and Brian W. J. Mahy of the Centers for Disease Control and Prevention, as quoted in Luis Villarreal, "Are Viruses Alive," *Scientific American*, December 2004, p. 98.

Chapter 4: The Havoc

Birgit Winther's study can be found in B. Winther et al., "Light and scanning electron microscopy of nasal biopsy material from patients with naturally acquired colds," *Acta Otolaryngol* 97 (3-4): 309-18 (1984). As Jack Gwaltney Jr. describes it, a biopsy of nasal epithelial cells infected with rhinovirus was initially conducted by Robert Crouch and his group at NIAID, but the group considered the experiment a bust. See R. G. J. Douglas, "Pathogenesis of rhinovirus common colds in human volunteers," *Ann Otol Rhino Laryngol* 79: 563-71 (1970). See also B. Winther et al., "Sites of rhinovirus recovery after point inoculation of the upper airway," *J Am Med*

Assoc 256: 1763-7 (1986). A study revealing the small number of cells that showed signs of replicating virus is found in R. B. Turner et al., "Shedding of infected epithelial cells in rhinovirus colds," *J Infect Dis* 145 (6): 849-53 (1982).

For the theory on the genesis of cold symptoms, see J. Owen Hendley, "The host response, not the virus, causes the symptoms of the common cold," *Clin Infect Dis* 26: 847-8 (1998).

The quotation from Marion Nestle about Kellogg's claims for its Cocoa Krispies can be found at www.foodpolitics.com/?s=cocoa+krispies. Information about children's runny noses comes from N. Mygind et al., "The common cold and asthma," *Allergy* 54 (Suppl 57): 146-59 (1999). Margaret Visser's quotation about mucus is found in her book *The Way We Are* (Faber and Faber, 1996), p. 164.

The description of Steven Churchill's work on the evolution of the nose comes from an interview with Churchill in 2005. His research appears in S. E. Churchill et al., "Morphological variation and airflow dynamics in the human nose," *Am J Hum Biol* 16: 625-38 (2004). Ron Eccles's study on nasal shape appears in S. C. Leong and R. Eccles, "A systematic review of the nasal index and the significance of the shape and size of the nose in rhinology," *Clin Otolaryngol* 34 (3): 191-8 (2009). Jack Gwaltney Jr.'s study on sinuses can be found in J. M. Gwaltney et al., "Computed tomographic study of the common cold," *New Eng J Med* 330 (1): 25-30 (1994).

The line from Ogden Nash occurs in the poem "Can I get you a glass of water?" *New Yorker*, March 28, 1953. The "Talk of the Town" story, written by Ruth C. Woodman and St. Clair McKelway, appears in "Cousin Caddie," *New Yorker*, June 10, 1961, p. 27, available at: www.newyorker.com/archive/1961/06/10/1961_06_10_027_TNY_CARDS_000267043#ixzz0dNIAWSnb. Information on cough frequency can be found in J. J. Kuhn et al., "Antitussive effect of guaifenesin in young adults with natural colds," *Chest* 82: 713-18 (1982). The quotation from Phil Jones comes from a response on October 11, 2007, to the NOSE email discussion group, conducted by Ron Eccles.

James Lovelock's story about the crewmen of the B-17 bombers comes from Lovelock (2000), p. 82. The term "Valsalva maneuver" is named for Antonio Maria Valsalva, a 17th-century anatomist from Bologna, who first coined the term "eustachian tube" and investigated other parts of the human ear. For advice on flying with colds and other illnesses, see "Medical guidelines for air travel," *Aviation Space and Environ Med* 74 (5), Section II Supplement (2003).

Gay Talese's famous profile of Frank Sinatra was published in *Esquire* in April 1966. The impact of colds on mood is explored in M. Schaechter, "Demeanors, moods, and microbes," *Microbe* 1 (8): 348–49 (2006). Denise Janicki-Deverts's research appears in D. Janicki-Deverts et al., "Infection-induced proinflammatory cytokines are associated with decreases in positive affect, but not increases in negative affect," *Brain Beh Imm* 21: 301–7 (2007). The effects of colds on performance are addressed in A. Smith et al., "Effects of the common cold on subjective alertness, reaction time, and eye movements," *J Psychophysiology* 13 (3): 145–51 (1999); A. Smith, "Effects of the common cold on mood and performance," *Psychoneuroendocrinology* 23 (7): 733–9 (1998); A. P. Smith, "Respiratory virus infections and performance," *Phil Trans R Soc Lond B* 327: 519–28 (1990); A. P. Smith, "A review of the effects of colds and influenza on human performance," *Occupational Medicine* 39: 65–68 (1989).

Research on the effect of colds on running and other forms of exercise can be found in T. G. Weidner et al., "Effects of viral upper respiratory illness on running gait," *Athletic Training* 32: 309–14 (1997); T. G. Weidner et al., "Pilot study: effects of viral upper respiratory illness on physical performance," *Sport Med* 15: 21–5 (1998).

Studies on the effects of colds on reasoning, learning, and memory can be found in R. S. Bucks et al., "Selective effects of upper respiratory tract infection on cognition, mood and emotion processing: A prospective study," *Brain Beh Immun* 22: 399–407 (2008).

A study on the link between cytokines and malaise and other sickness behaviors occurs in K. W. Kelley, "Cytokine-induced sickness behavior," *Brain Beh Immun* 17 Suppl 1: S112–8 (2003). See also J. McAfoose and B. T. Baune, "Evidence for a cytokine model of cognitive function," *Neurosci and Biobehav Rev* 33 (3): 355–66 (2008).

Drake's study of the impact of colds on sleep and alertness occurs in C. L. Drake et al., "Effects of an experimentally induced rhinovirus cold on sleep, performance, and daytime alertness," *Physiol Behav* 71: 75–81 (2000).

A description of Jack Gwaltney Jr.'s study on asymptomatic infection appears in J. M. Gwaltney, "Rhinoviruses," in A. S. Evans and R. A. Kaslow, eds., *Viral Infection of Humans: Epidemiology and Control*, 4th ed. (New York City: Plenum Press, 1997), pp. 815–38.

Chapter 5: The Terrain

Studies on children's hand-to-mouth episodes appear in N. S. Tulve et al., "Frequency of mouthing behavior in young children," *J Exposure Analysis and Environ Epidem* 12: 259-64 (2002). Harley Rotbart's quotation about day care occurs in Rotbart (2008), p. 43.

Information on the link between temperature and colds can be found in R. G. J. Douglas et al., "Exposure to cold environment and rhinovirus common cold: Failure to demonstrate effect," *New Engl J Med* 279: 742-7 (1968). Ron Eccles's study on foot-chilling and cold incidence appears in C. Johnson and R. Eccles, "Acute cooling of the feet and the onset of common cold symptoms," *Family Practice* 22: 608-13 (2005).

The Exeter study appears in F. Sargent et al., "Further studies on stability of resistance to the common cold: The importance of constitution," *AJH* 45: 29-32 (1947). The Seattle Virus Watch study occurs in J. P. Fox et al., "The Seattle Virus Watch V. Epidemiologic observations of rhinovirus infections, 1965-1969, in families with young children," *Am J Epidemiol* 101 (2): 122-43 (1975). Reports on the Exeter study and Thomas Ball's investigations can be found in T. Ball et al., "Is there a common cold constitution?" *Ambulatory Pediatrics* 2 (4): 261-7 (2002); and T. Ball et al., "Influence of attendance at day care on the common cold from birth through 13 years of age," *Arch Pediatr Adolesc Med* 156 (2): 121-6 (2002).

Sheldon Cohen's research on the effects of sleep disruption and deprivation on susceptibility can be found in S. Cohen et al., "Sleep habits and susceptibility to the common cold," *Arch Intern Med* 169 (1): 62-7 (2009). The study of sleep and inflammation occurs in S. R. Patel et al., "Sleep duration and biomarkers of inflammation," *Sleep* 32 (2): 200-4 (2009).

For an excellent discussion of stress, both acute and chronic, see Bruce McEwen, *The End of Stress as We Know It* (Washington, D.C.: Dana Press, 2002). David Tyrrell's comment on the value of stress studies can be found in Tyrrell (2002), p. 209. Cohen's studies on stress, socioeconomic status, emotional style, and cold susceptibility appear in S. Cohen et al., "Objective and subjective socioeconomic status and susceptibility to the common cold," *Health Psychology* 27 (2): 268-74 (2008); S. Cohen et al., "Positive emotional style predicts resistance to illness after experimental exposure to rhinovirus or influenza A virus," *Psychosomatic Med* 68: 809-815 (2006); "Emotional style, nasal cytokines, and illness expression after experimental rhinovirus exposure," *Brain Beh Imm* 20: 175-81 (2006);

S. D. Pressman and S. Cohen, "Does positive affect influence health?" *Psych Bull* 131 (6): 925-71; S. Cohen et al., "Childhood socioeconomic status and host resistance to infectious illness in adulthood," *Psychosomatic Med* 66: 553-8 (2004); S. Cohen et al., "Emotional style and susceptibility to the common cold," *Psychosomatic Med* 65: 652-7 (2003); S. Cohen, "Types of stressors that increase susceptibility to the common cold in healthy adults," *Health Psychology* 17 (3): 214-23 (1998); S. Cohen, "Negative life events, perceived stress, negative affect, and susceptibility to the common cold," *J Pers and Soc Psych* 64 (1): 131-40 (1993); S. Cohen et al., "Psychological stress and susceptibility to the common cold," *New Engl J Med* 325 (9): 606-12 (1991). His work on the influence of alcohol and cigarettes can be found in S. Cohen et al., "Smoking, alcohol consumption, and susceptibility to the common cold," *Am J Public Health* 83 (9): 1277-83 (1993).

Charles Matthews's study on exercise and cold susceptibility occurs in C. E. Matthews, "Moderate to vigorous physical activity and influence on upper-respiratory tract infection," *Med Sci Sports Exer* 34 (8): 1242-8 (2002). The research on exercise, colds, and menopausal women can be found in J. Chubak, "Moderate-intensity exercise reduces the incidence of colds among postmenopausal women," *Am J Med* 119: 938-43 (2006). Evidence of the negative effects of extreme exercise appears in L. T. Mackinnon, "Chronic exercise training effects on immune function," *Med Sci Sports Exerc* 32 (7 Suppl): S369-76 (2000). For Ad Vingerhoets's study on leisure sickness, see G. L. Van Heck and A. J. J. M. Vingerhoets, "Leisure sickness: A biopsychosocial perspective," *Psych Topics* 16 (2): 187-200 (2007). Cohen's work on social ties occurs in S. Cohen et al., "Sociability and susceptibility to the common cold," *Psych Sci* 14 (5): 389-95 (2003); and S. Cohen et al., "Social ties and susceptibility to the common cold," *J Am Med Assoc* 277 (24): 1940-4 (1997).

Chapter 6: Killer Colds

My account of Paige Villers's illness and the outbreak of adenovirus 14 is drawn from the CDC's *Morb Mort Weekly Rep* 56 (45): 1181-4; and from Louis Arana-Barradas, "Michelle's Yellow Rose," *Airman Magazine,* March/April 2008: pp. 10-14. The evolutionary handshake between virulence and transmission is discussed in "Evolution from a virus's view," December 2007, at www.evolution.berkeley.edu.

For a general discussion of the role of rhinoviruses in other illnesses, see R. B. Turner, "Rhinovirus: More than just a common cold virus," *J Infect*

Dis 195: 765-6 (2007). N. G. Papadopoulus and S. L. Johnston, "The rhinovirus—not such an innocent?" *Q J Med* 94: 1-3 (2001). The study using new molecular detection techniques to reveal the role of rhinoviruses in asthma is found in E. K. Miller, "Rhinovirus-associated hospitalization in young children," *J Infect Dis* 195 (6): 773-81 (2007).

Sebastian Johnston's research appears in N. W. Bartlett et al., "Mouse models of rhinovirus-induced disease and exacerbation of allergic airway inflammation," *Nature Medicine* 14: 199-204 (2008); S. D. Message et al., "Rhinovirus-induced lower respiratory illness is increased in asthma and related to virus load and Th1/2 cytokine and Il-10 production," *Proc Natl Acad Sci* 105 (36): 13562-67 (2008); S. L. Johnston, "Innate immunity in the pathogenesis of virus-induced asthma exacerbations," *Proc Am Thorac Soc* 4: 267-70 (2007); P. A. Wark et al., "Asthmatic bronchial epithelial cells have a deficient innate immune response to infection with rhinovirus," *J Exp Med* 201 (6): 937-47 (2005); and S. D. Message and S. L. Johnston, "Viruses in asthma," *Br Med Bull* 61: 29-43 (2002).

Discussions of the hygiene hypothesis occur in W. O. Cookson and M. F. Moffatt, "Asthma—an epidemic in the absence of infection," *Science* 275 (5296): 41-2 (1997); S. L. Johnston and P. J. M. Openshaw, "The protective effect of childhood infections," *Br Med J* 322: 376-7 (2001); and S. Illi et al., "Early childhood infectious diseases and the development of asthma up to school age: a birth cohort study," *Br Med J* 322: 390-5 (2001). For the theory on the role played by mild rhinovirus infections in developing effective antiviral defenses, see J. Yoo et al., "Microbial manipulation of immune function for asthma prevention. Inferences from clinical trials," *Proc Am Thoracic Soc* 4: 277-82 (2007). For a discussion of the link between antibiotics and asthma, see Rotbart (2008), p. 156.

Chapter 7: To Kill a Cold

My account of the chlorine chamber capers draws on a fascinating chapter by David Nader and Spasoje Marčinko, "The rise and fall of 'chlorine chambers' against cold and flu," in Hasok Chang and Catherine Jackson, eds., *An Element of Controversy: The Life of Chlorine in Science, Medicine, Technology and War* (British Society for the History of Science, 2007); Russell (2001), especially p. 63; and E. B. Vedder and H. P. Sawyer, "Chlorin [sic] as a therapeutic agent in certain respiratory diseases," *J Am Med Assoc* 82: 764-66 (1924). Reference to observations linking chlorine workers with freedom from colds and flu occurs in the article "Chlorine," in *Time* magazine, December 8, 1924. Edward Vedder's research on, and promotion of, chlorine gas therapy can be found in E. B. Vedder, "The present status of chlorine gas therapy," *Trans Am Climatolog Clin Assoc* 41: 203–16 (1925); "Recent development with regard to chlorine treatment of certain respiratory diseases," *J Med Soc New Jersey* 22: 40 (1925); and "Chlorine gas therapy," *Ann Clin Med* 4: 21 (1925). The newspaper quotation about the new fashion of chlorine treatment is found in George Rothwell Brown, "Post-scripts," *Washington Post*, May 29, 1924, p. 1. Vedder's quotation about the prophylactic possibilities of chlorine can be found in Vedder (1925), p. 303. Russell's description of the role of chlorine treatment in refurbishing the image of chlorine appears in Russell (2001), p. 63. The physician's quotation on the inefficacy of chlorine for cold treatment occurs in Russell (2001), p. 63.

Descriptions of historical treatments for colds can be found in J. M. Gwaltney, "Viral respiratory infection therapy: Historical perspectives and current trials," *Am J Med* 112 (6A): 33S–41S (2002); "Developing treatments: The common cold," Museum of the Royal Pharmaceutical Society of Great Britain, available at www.rpsgb.org/pdfs/mussheetcold.pdf. The *Scientific American* reference to borax treatment in 1895 occurs in *Scientific American*, May 1995, p. 10. The statistics on NIH funding for cold research come from the press office at NCCAM (emailed January 15, 2010). The quotation about the general practitioner comes from Dr. Marshall Marinker, as quoted in Worrall (2006), p. 123. The 2008 survey on the use of cough and cold medications for children can be found in L. Vernacchio et al., "Cough and cold medication use by U.S. children, 1999–2006: results from the Slone survey," *Pediatrics* 122 (2): e323–9 (2008).

For information on over-the-counter cold medications and other treatments, M. Simasek and D. A. Blandino, "Treatment of the common cold," *Am Fam Phys* 75 (4): 515–20; P. S. Muether and J. M. Gwaltney, "Variant effect of first- and second-generation antihistamines as clues to their mechanism of action on the sneeze reflex in the common cold," *Clin Infect Dis* 33: 1483–8 (2001); B. Winther and N. Mygind, "The therapeutic effectiveness of ibuprofen on the symptoms of naturally acquired common colds," *Am J Rhinolog* 15 (4): 239–42 (2001); R. Eccles, "Efficacy and safety of over-the-counter analgesics in the treatment of cold and flu," *J Clin Pharm Ther* 31 (4): 309–19 (2006); D. Taverner and J. Latte, "Nasal decongestants for the common cold," *Cochrane Database Syst Rev* 2007 (19): CCD001953; A. I. M. Sutter et al., "Antihistamines for the common cold,"

Cochrane Database Syst Rev 2003 (3): CD 001267; S. M. Smith, "Over-the-counter medications for acute cough in children and adults in ambulatory settings," *Cochrane Database Syst Rev* 2008 (1): CD001831.

Reports of the dangers of over-the-counter cold and cough medications for children can be found in R. C. Dart et al., "Pediatric fatalities associated with over the counter (nonprescription) cough and cold medications," *Ann Emerg Med* 53 (4): 411–7 (2009). See also J. M. Sharfstein et al., "Over the counter but no longer under the radar—pediatric cough and cold medications," *New Engl J Med* 357: 2321–4 (2009).

Quotations from Stephen Rennard on the motivation for his experiment on chicken soup come from the University of Nebraska Medical Center press release, dated October 21, 2008 (www.unmc.edu/chickensoup/newsrelease.htm) and from email correspondence with Dr. Rennard. The study itself occurs in S. Rennard, "Chicken soup inhibits neutrophil chemotaxis in vitro," *Chest* 118: 1150–7 (2000). The quotation from Rennard's colleague is found in the UNMC press release cited above. The quotation from the two enthusiastic chicken soup fans appears in A. Ohry and J. Tsafrir, "Is chicken soup an essential drug?" *J Can Med Assoc* 161 (12): 1532–3 (1999).

Information on vitamin C can be found in REFS and A. Strohle and A. Hahn, "Vitamin C and immune function," *Med Mnatsschr Pharm* 32 (2): 49–54 (2009).

Gwaltney's review on zinc appears in T. J. Caruso et al., "Treatment of naturally acquired common colds with zinc," *Clin Infect Dis* 45 (5): 569–74 (2007). It should be noted that George Eby maintains that the failure of zinc lozenges currently on the market to show any effect is due to their composition, containing insufficient amounts of positively charged, ionic zinc. See G. A. Eby, "Zinc lozenges as cure for the common cold—A review and hypothesis," *Medical Hypotheses*, Nov. 9, 2009.

Statistics on the use of alternative treatments for colds comes from P. M. Barnes et al., "Complementary and alternative medicine use among adults: United States, 2002," *Advance Data from Vital and Health Statistics* 343, 1–19 (Hyattsville, Maryland: National Center for Health Statistics, 2004); D. W. Kaufman, "Recent patterns of medication use in the ambulatory adult population of the U.S.," *J Am Med Assoc* 287: 337–44 (2002). See also the page on alternative common cold medications on the website of the Common Cold Centre: www.cardiff.ac.uk/biosi/subsites/cold/alt.html.

Rotbart's discussion of alternative therapies appears in Rotbart

NOTES

(2008), p. 310. Turner's evaluation of the current state of herbal treatment research can be found in R. B. Turner, "Clinical trials of herbal treatments," *Evaluation & the Health Professions* 32 (4): 410–16 (2009); and R. B. Turner, "Studies of 'natural' remedies for the common cold: pitfalls and pratfalls," *CMAJ* 173 (9) (2005).

A description of Native Americans' use of echinacea can be found in Daniel Moerman, *Native American Ethnobotany* (Timber Press, 1998). The recent review of echinacea's efficacy in treating colds occurs in S. A. Shah et al., "Evaluation of echinacea for the prevention and treatment of the common cold: a meta-analysis," *Lancet* 7: 473–80 (2007). Turner's 2005 review occurs in R. B. Turner et al., "An evaluation of *Echinacea angustifolia* in experimental rhinovirus infection," *New Eng J Med* 353 (4): 341–8 (2005).

My account of the Airborne story draws from the class action suit of *David Wilson v. Airborne*, downloaded from http://cspinet.org/new/pdf/airbornecomplaint.pdf; the Airborne settlement website at www.airbornehealthsettlement.com/index.htm; FTC press release August 14, 2008, "Makers of airborne settle FTC charges of deceptive advertising," downloaded May 20, 2009, from www.ftc.gov/opa/2008/08/airborne.shtm; and the ABC story, reported in "Does Airborne Really Stave off Colds?," February 27, 2006, available at http://abcnews.go.com/GMA/OnCall/story?id=1664514&page=1.

The Federal Trade Commission comment was delivered by Lydia Parnes, director of the FTC's Bureau of Consumer protection.

Information on Zicam and its maker Matrixx can be found on the Matrixx website, www.matrixxinc.com; and S. G. Boodman, "Paying through the nose," *Washington Post,* January 31, 2006: HE01. Berkowitz's comment on Zicam occurs on his blog, "The way I work," at www.inc.com/magazine/20080701/the-way-i-work-roger-berkowitz_pagen_2.html. Matrixx's response to the FDA recommendations is revealed in a full-page advertisement in the *New York Times,* June 22, 2009, p. A5.

Information on COLD-FX and its maker, Afexa, is found at the COLD-FX website: www.COLD-FXusa.com; J. K. Seida et al., "North American (*Panax quinquefolius*) and Asian ginseng (*Panax ginseng*) preparations for prevention of the common cold in healthy adults: A systematic review," *Complementary and Altern Med*, published online July 10, 2009: eCAM, doi:10.1093/ecam/nep068; A. Nguyen and V. Slavik, "COLD-FX," *Can Fam Phys* 53: 481–2 (2007); D. Baines, "Hard to swallow: CV technologies," *Canadian Business*, March 27–April 9, 2006. The description of the tray-table advertising effort is drawn from a story by Stephanie Clifford in

Inc. Magazine, July 2007. The 2008 COLD-FX study is described in a press release issued by Afexa on September 15, 2008.

Discussion of placebo can be found in Ron Eccles, "The power of placebo," *Curr Allergy Asthma Rep* 7: 100–4 (2007); A. K. Vallance, "Something out of nothing: the placebo effect," *Adv Psych Treat* 12: 287–296 (2006). Ron Eccles's comment on placebo occurs in Kathryn Senior, "Alternative medicine and the cold challenge," *Lancet* 352: 1685 (1998). The Thomas Jefferson and Richard Cabot quotations appear in A. J. M de Craen et al., "Placebos and placebo effects in medicine: historical overview," *J Roy Soc Med* 92: 511–15 (1999). The study on the impact of product cost on the placebo effect appears in "Commercial features of placebo and therapeutic efficacy," *J Am Med Assoc* 299 (9): 1016–7 (2008). Research on the impact of drug color on the placebo effect occurs in A. J. M. de Craen et al., "Effect of colour of drugs: systematic review of perceived effect of drugs and their effectiveness," *Br Med J* 313: 1624–6 (1996). Harold Diehl's study on placebo and common cold occurs in H. Diehl, "Medicinal treatment of the common cold," *J Am Med Assoc* 101: 2042–49 (1933). Ron Eccles's study on placebo effect and cough treatment appears in R. Eccles, "Importance of placebo effect in cough clinical trials," *Lung,* Sept. 16, 2009; and P. C. L. Lee et al., "The antitussive effect of placebo treatment on cough associated with acute upper respiratory infection," *Psychosomatic Med* 67: 314–7 (2005).

The investigation of genetic drift and the genetic codes for rhinoviruses appears in A. L. Kistler, "Genome-wide diversity and selective pressure in the human rhinovirus," *Virol J* 4: 40 (2007).

Research on potential cold cures can be found in W. G. Nichols et al., "Respiratory viruses other than influenza virus: impact and therapeutic advances," *Clin Microb Rev* 21 (2): 274–90 (2008); A. K. Patick, "Rhinovirus chemotherapy," *Antiviral Res* 72 (2-3): 391–6 (2006); F. G. Hayden et al., "Efficacy and safety of oral pleconaril for treatment of colds due to picornaviruses in adults," *Clin Infect Dis* 36 (12): 1523–32 (2003); and R. B. Turner, "Efficacy of tremacamra, a soluble intercellular adhesion molecule 1 for experimental rhinovirus infection: a randomized clinical trial," *J Am Med Assoc* 281 (19): 1797–804 (1999). Jack Gwaltney Jr.'s study on antiviral /anti-inflammatory treatment appears in J. M. Gwaltney, "Combined antiviral-antimediator treatment for the common cold," *J Infect Dis* 186: 147–54 (2002). A new study on a potential target for a cold vaccine appears in U. Katpally et al., "Antibodies to the buried N terminus of rhinovirus VP4 exhibit cross-serotypic neutralization," *J Virology* 83 (14): 7040–8 (2009). The 2009 study on the effect of empathy on the common cold occurs in

D. P. Rakel, "Practitioner empathy and the duration of the common cold," *Fam Med* 41 (7): 494–501 (2009).

Chapter 8: Don't Catch Me If You Can

Donald Trump's comment on shaking hands appears on his blog at www.trumpuniversity.com/blog/post/2008/07/the-importance-of-a-good -handshake.cfm.

Spike Wing Sing Lee's study on sneezing can be found in S. W. S. Lee, "Sneezing in time of a flu pandemic: Public sneezing increases perception of unrelated risks and shifts preference for federal spending," *Psychological Science*, November 9, 2009.

The studies of face mask use appear in J. L. Jacobs et al., "Use of surgical face masks to reduce the incidence of the common cold among health care workers in Japan: a randomized controlled trial," *Am J Infect Control* 37 (5): 417–9 (2009). My account of the 2009 Ig Nobel ceremony is drawn from the *Br Med J* 339: b4089 (2009). The story of Ignac Semmelweis is described in M. Best and D. Neuhauser, "Ignaz Semmelweis and the birth of infection control," *Qual Saf Health Care* 1: 233–4 (2004); the Semmelweis Society International website: www.semmelweis.org; and Irvine London, *The Tragedy of Childbed Fever* (Oxford, 2000). The study on Operation Stop Cough appears in M. A. K Ryan et al., "Handwashing and respiratory illness among young adults in military training," *Am J Prev Med* 21 (2): 79–83 (2001). Rotbart's comments on soap and dry hands appear in Rotbart (2008), p. 270. Elaine Larson's work on the efficacy of various cleaning products and other aspects of cold prevention occurs in A. E. Aiello et al., "Effect of hand hygiene on infectious disease risk in the community setting: A meta-analysis," *Am J Public Health* 98 (8): 1372–81 (2008); S. F. Bloomfield et al., "The effectiveness of hand hygiene procedures in reducing the risks of infections in home and community settings including handwashing and alcohol-based hand sanitizers," *Am J Infect Control* 35 (10): S27–S64 (2007); A. E. Aiello et al., "Consumer antibacterial soaps: Effective or just risky?" *Clin Infect Dis* 45 (Suppl 2): S137–47 (2007); E. L. Larson, "Warned, but not well armed: preventing viral upper respiratory infections in households," *Public Health Nursing* 24 (1): 48–59 (2006); and E. L. Larson, "Effect of antibacterial home cleaning and handwashing products on infectious disease symptoms," *Ann Int Med* 140 (5): 321–29 (2004). Surveys on Americans' hand-washing habits appear in the report on the American Society for Microbiology Survey on washing hands at airports, dated September 15, 2003, available at http://asm.org/media /index.asp?bid=217; Soap and Detergent Association's 2007 survey; and the GOJO "Germ" Survey, May 2004. Reports of studies on peer pressure and other influences on hand-washing habits appear in E. Scott and K. Vanick, "A survey of hand hygiene practices on a residential college campus," *Am J Infect Control* 35 (10): 694–6 (2007); E. L. Larson, "Hand hygiene behavior in a pediatric emergency department and a pediatric intensive care unit: comparison of use of 2 dispenser systems," *Am J Crit Care* 14 (4): 304–11 (2005); and the Water and Sanitation Program website: www. wsp.org. Elaine Larson's study of misconceptions about colds appears in "Knowledge and misconceptions regarding upper respiratory infections and influenza among urban Hispanic households: Need for targeted messaging," *J Immig Min Health* 11: 71–82 (2009). Accounts of the "Catch it, Bin it, Kill it" campaign can be found at the U.K. Department of Health website: www.dh.gov.uk. Information on the "gross messaging" study appears in "University of Denver uses 'gross' messaging to increases hand-washing, fight norovirus," at www.eurekalert.org/pub_releases/2008-12/ uod-uod121508.php. Ron Turner's studies on hand sanitizers occur in R. B. Turner et al., "Efficacy of organic acids in hand cleansers for prevention of rhinovirus infections," *Antimicrob Agents and Chemother* 48 (7): 2595–8 (2004); R. B. Turner and J. O. Hendley, "Virucidal hand treatments for prevention of rhinovirus infection," *J Antimicrob Chemother* 56: 805–7 (2005); R. B. Turner et al., "Effectiveness of hand sanitizers with and without organic acids for removal of rhinovirus from hands," *Antimicrob Agents Chemother*, January 4, 2010.

Rotbart's comment on the Japanese practice of *ojigi* appears in Rotbart (2008), p. 268. The study on training children not to self-inoculate appears in D. L. Corley et al., "Prevention of postinfectious asthma in children by reducing self-inoculatory behavior," *J Pediatr Psychol* 12: 519–31 (1987). The 2008 survey on sick leave was a poll conducted by National Public Radio, the Kaiser Family Foundation, and the Harvard School of Public Health May 24–June 8, 2008. Blendon is quoted in the report on NPR's *Morning Edition*, July 28, 2008. See also a report on a study of "presenteeism" by researchers at Cornell University Institute for Health and Productivity Studies (IHPS) in a press release dated April 20, 2004, available at www .news.cornell.edu/releases/April04/cost.illness.jobs.sssl.html.

Chapter 9: In Defense of Colds

My discussion of virulence and the adaptations of cold viruses draws on Kirchberger (2007), p. 8; S. Dreschers, "The cold case: are rhinoviruses perfectly adapted pathogens?" *Cell Mol Life Sci* 64 (2): 181–91 (2007); J. Lederberg, "Emerging infections: An evolutionary perspective," *Emerg Infect Dis* 4 (3): (1998); and "Evolution from a virus's view," December 2007, at www.evolution.berkeley.edu.

Information on the possible role of rhinovirus in affecting the spread of influenza can be found in J. S. Casalengo et al., "Rhinoviruses delayed the circulation of pandemic influenza (H1N1) 2009 Virus in France," *Clin Microbiol Infect,* Jan. 28, 2010; A. Linde et al., "Does viral interference affect spread of influenza?" *Euro Surveill* 14 (40): pii=19354 (2009); R. M. Greer et al., "Do rhinoviruses reduce the probability of viral co-detection during acute respiratory tract infections," *J Clin Virol* 45 (1): 10–5 (2009).

Studies on the use of cold viruses in therapies for other diseases can be found in G. F. Arnold et al., "Broad neutralization of human immunodeficiency virus type 1 (HIV-1) elicited from human rhinoviruses that display the HIV-1 gp41 ELDKWA Epitope," *J Virology* 83 (10): 5087–5100 (2009); and L. Zhang et al., "CFTR delivery to 25% of surface epithelial cells restores normal rates of mucus transport to human cystic fibrosis airway epithelium," *PLoS Biol* Jul. 7 (7) 2009.

Luis Villarreal's perspective on viruses appears in "Can viruses make us human?" *Proc Am Phil Soc* 148 (3): 296 (2003); and L. P. Villarreal, "Are Viruses Alive?" *Scientific American,* December 2004, pp. 98–101. The quotation from Lewis Thomas occurs in *The Lives of a Cell* (Penguin, 1978). Research on endogenous retroviruses appears in Robin A. Weiss, "The discovery of endogenous retroviruses," *Retrovirology* 3: 67 (2006).

Appendix: Cold Comforts

For a review of the impact of NSAIDs on the common cold, see S. Y. Kim, "Non-steroidal anti-inflammatory drugs for the common cold," *Cochrane Database of Syst Rev* 2009 (3): CD005362. The evidence for the undesirable effects of certain pain relievers on colds can be found in N. M. Graham et al., "Adverse effects of aspirin, acetaminophen, and ibuprofen on immune function, viral shedding, and clinical status in rhinovirus-infected volunteers," *J Infect Dis* 162: 1277–82 (1990). The review on antihistamines occurs in A. I. M. De Sutter et al., "Antihistamines for the common cold," *Cochrane Database of Syst Rev* 2006 (4). For a review of the efficacy of various cough treatments, see Z. C. Boujaoude and M. R. Pratter, "Clinical approaches to acute cough," *Lung*, August 22, 2009.

The survey on how mothers from different cultures treat colds can be found in L. M. Pachter et al., "Home-based therapies for the common cold among European American and ethnic minority families," *Arch Pediatr Adolesc Med* 152: 1083–8 (1998). Bruce Barrett's study on people's expectations of benefit from cold remedies appears in B. Barrett et al., "Sufficiently important difference for common cold: Severity reduction," *Ann Fam Med* 5 (4): 216–23 (2007).

Jack Gwaltney Jr.'s review of zinc appears in T. J. Caruso, C. G. Prober, and J. M. Gwaltney, "Treatment of naturally acquired common colds with zinc," *Clin Infect Dis* 45 (5): 569–74 (2007). For information on COLD-FX, see references listed in chapter 7. The 2005 study occurs in Gerald N. Predy, Vinti Goel, Ray Lovlin, Allan Donner, Larry Stitt, Tapan K. Basu, "Efficacy of an extract of North American ginseng containing poly-furanosyl-pyranosyl-saccharides for preventing upper respiratory tract infections: a randomized controlled trial," *Can Med Assoc J* 173 (9): 1043–8 (2005). Reviews on the efficacy of echinacea appear in L. K. Barrett et al., "Echinacea for preventing and treating the common cold (review)," *Coch Lib* 2006 (1): 1–39; S. A. Shah et al., "Evaluation of echinacea for the prevention and treatment of the common cold: a meta-analysis," *Lancet* 7: 473–80 (2007). Turner's 2005 review occurs in R. B. Turner et al., "An evaluation of *Echinacea angustifolia* in experimental rhinovirus infection," *New Eng J Med* 353 (4): 341–8 (2005). Information on the effects of exercise on cold susceptibility, duration, and severity can be found in T. Weidner, "Effect of exercise on upper respiratory tract infection in sedentary subjects," *Br J Sports Med* 37: 304–6 (2003). The recent review of garlic occurs in E. Lissiman et al., "Garlic for the common cold," *Cochrane Database of Syst Rev* 2009, Issue 3. Art. No. CD006206. The latest review of ginseng appears in J. K. Seida et al., "North American (*Panax quinquefolius*) and Asian ginseng (*Panax ginseng*) preparations for prevention of the common cold in healthy adults: A systematic review," *Complementary and Altern Med*, published online July 10, 2009: eCAM, doi:10.1093/ecam/nep068. The study on the effects of honey on cough occurs in I. M. Paul, "Effect of honey, dextromethorphan, and no treatment on nocturnal cough and sleep quality for coughing children and their parents," *Arch Pediatr Adolesc Med* 161 (12): 1140–6 (2007). The

NOTES

2007 study on hot drinks appears in A. Sanu, "The effects of a hot drink on nasal airflow and symptoms of common cold and flu," *Rhinology* 46 (4): 271–5 (2008). The report on clinical trials on the effects of humidified air appears in M. Singh, "Heated, humidified air for the common cold," *Cochrane Database Syst Rev* 2006 (3): CD001728. Research on nasal washing can be found in I. Šlapak, "Efficacy of isotonic nasal wash (seawater) in the treatment and prevention of rhinitis in children," *Arch Otolaryngol Head Neck Surg* 134 (1): 67–74 (2008). The research on saline is found in J. E. Gern, "Inhibition of rhinovirus replication in vitro and in vivo by acid-buffered saline," *J Infec Dis* 195: 1137–43 (2007). The studies of probiotics appear in M. De Vrese et al., "Probiotic bacteria reduced duration and severity but not the incidence of common cold episodes in a double blind, randomized, controlled trial," *Vaccine* 24 (44–46): 6670–4 (2006); K. Hatakka et al., "Effect of long term consumption of a probiotic milk on the infections in children attending day care centres: double-blind, randomised trial," *Brit Med J* 322: 1327–9 (2001); and in P. Winkler, "Effect of a dietary supplement containing probiotic bacteria plus vitamins and minerals on common cold infections and cellular immune parameters," *Int J Clin Pharmacol Ther* 43 (7): 318–26 (2005). Research on saline nasal sprays can be found in P. Adam et al., "A clinical trial of hypertonic saline nasal spray in subjects with the common cold or rhinosinusitis," *Arch Fam Med* 7: 39–43(1998). The review of the effects of steaming on the common cold appears in M. Singh, "Heated, humidified air for the common cold," *Cochrane Database of Syst Rev* 2006, Issue 3. Art. No.: CD001728. The Dutch study on the effects of eating on interferon levels occurs in G. R. Van den Brink, "Feed a cold, starve a fever," *Clin Diagn Lab Immunol* 9 (1): 182–3 (2002). The research on the impact of empathy on the common cold occurs in D. P. Rakel, "Practitioner empathy and the duration of the common cold," *Fam Med* 41 (7): 494–501 (2009). The 2009 study on the effects of Vicks VapoRub on children appears in J. C. Abanses et al., "Vicks VapoRub induces mucin secretion, decreases ciliary beat frequency, and increases tracheal mucus transport in the ferret trachea," *Chest* 135 (1): 143–8 (2009). Investigations of the impact of vitamin C on the common cold appear in H. Hemilä, "Vitamin C for preventing and treating the common cold," *Cochrane Database of Syst Rev* 18 (3): CD000980 (2004); H. Hemilä, "Vitamin C and common cold incidence. A review of studies with subjects under heavy physical stress," *Int J Sports Med* 17: 379–83 (1996). The epidemiological study of vitamin D and colds occurs in A. A. Ginde et al., "Association between serum 25-hydroxyvitamin D level and upper respiratory tract infection in the Third National Health and Nutrition Examination Survey," *Arch Int Med* 169 (4): 384 (2009). The reviews on zinc occur in T. J. Caruso et al., "Treatment of naturally acquired common colds with zinc," *Clin Infect Dis* Sep 1; 45 (5): 569–74 (2007); R. B. Turner, "Ineffectiveness of intranasal zinc gluconate for prevention of experimental rhinovirus colds," *Clin Infect Dis* 33: 1865–70 (2001); and R. B. Turner and W. E. Cetnarowski, "Effect of treatment with zinc gluconate or zinc acetate on experimental and natural colds," *Clin Infect Dis* 31: 1202–8 (2000). George Eby maintains that the failure of zinc lozenges currently on the market to show any effect is due to their composition, which contains insufficient amounts of positively charged, ionic zinc. See G. A. Eby, "Zinc lozenges as cure for the common cold—A review and hypothesis," *Medical Hypotheses*, Nov. 9, 2009.

The Jane Austen letters can be found online at www.jasna.org/pers uasions/printed/number12/kaplan.htm#4 and www.pemberley.com/jane info/brablet8.html#letter39.

The quotation about cold from Thomas Jefferson appears on the Monticello website: www.monticello.org/highlights/waistcoat.html. Apparently, the practice of foot soaking was widespread. Benjamin Rush, the medical adviser for the Lewis and Clark expedition, listed the cold foot soak as one of his "Rules for preserving good health," www.lewisandclarktrail .com/medical.htm. John Wesley, author of a popular book on curing diseases first published in 1747, recommended that parents protect their infants from colds by dipping them in cold water every morning until they reached nine months of age.

Charles Lamb's letter can be found at www.online-literature.com /lamb/best-letters/19/.

BIBLIOGRAPHY

Andrewes, Sir Christopher. *In Pursuit of the Common Cold*. London: William Heinemann Medical Books, 1973.

Boone, S. A., and C. P. Gerba. "Significance of fomites in the spread of respiratory and enteric viral disease," *App Envir Microbiology* 73 (6): 1687–96 (2007).

Bright, K. R., et al. "Occurrence of bacteria and viruses on elementary classroom surfaces and the potential role of classroom hygiene in the spread of infectious diseases," *Journal of School Nursing* 26 (1): 33–41 (2010).

Eccles, Ronald. "Mechanisms of symptoms of common cold and influenza," *Br J. Hosp Med* (Lond) 68 (2): 71–5 (2007).

Gerba, Charles P. "Application of quantitative risk assessment for formulating hygiene policy in the domestic setting," *Journal of Infection* 43: 92–8 (2001).

Gwaltney, J. M., Jr. "Life with rhinoviruses," in M. G. Ison et al., *Antiviral Research* 55: 228–78 (2002).

———. "Clinical significance and pathogenesis of viral respiratory infection," *Am J Med* 112 (6A): 13S–18S (2002).

Hayden, F. G. "Introduction: Emerging importance of rhinovirus," *Am J Med* 112 (6A): 1S–3S (2002).

Kirchberger, S., et al. "Modulation of the immune system by human rhinoviruses," *Int Arch Allergy Immunol* 142: 1–10 (2007).

Lovelock, James. *Homage to Gaia*. New York: Oxford University Press, 2000.

MacKay, Ian. "Human rhinoviruses: The cold wars resume," *J Clin Virology* 42: 297–320 (2008).

Monto, Arnold. "Epidemiology of viral respiratory infection," *Am J Med* 112 (6A): 4S–12S (2002).

Rotbart, Harley. *Germ Proof Your Kids.* Washington, D.C.: ASM Press, 2008.

Russell, Edmund. *War and Nature: Fighting Humans and Insects with Chemicals from World War I to Silent Spring.* New York: Cambridge University Press, 2001.

Tyrrell, David, and Michael Fielder. *Cold Wars: The Fight Against the Common Cold.* New York: Oxford University Press, 2002.

Vedder, E. B. "The present status of chlorine gas therapy," *Trans Am Climatolog Clin Assoc* 41: 203–216 (1925).

Worrall, Graham. *There's a Lot of It About: Acute Respiratory Infections in Primary Care.* Oxford: Radcliffe Publishing, 2006.

Websites

Common Cold Centre at Cardiff University, Wales: www.cf.ac.uk/biosi /subsites/cold/commoncold.html

University of Virginia: www.commoncold.org

INDEX

INDEX

INDEX

ABOUT THE AUTHOR

Although Jennifer Ackerman has been writing about health and science for the past 20 years, she still gets the average of two to four colds a year. Her most recent book, *Sex Sleep Eat Drink Dream: A Day in the Life of Your Body*, explores what goes on in the body over the course of a 24-hour day. The book was named a *New York Times* "Editor's Choice" and was supported by a fellowship in nonfiction from the National Endowment for the Arts. It has been published in ten languages. Ackerman is also the author of *Chance in the House of Fate: A Natural History of Heredity*, named a *New York Times* "New and Noteworthy" paperback and selected as a Library Journal Best Book of the Year. Her work on this book was supported by a fellowship from the Bunting Institute of Radcliffe College and a grant from the Alfred P. Sloan Foundation. In addition, Ackerman is the coauthor with Miriam Nelson of *The Strong Women's Guide to Total Health* (Rodale, 2010).

Ackerman's essays and articles have appeared in the *New York Times*, *National Geographic, More, Health, Real Simple, Women's Health*, and many other publications. She has written about subjects ranging from the importance of napping to food safety and the nature of dyslexia. Her writing has been collected in several anthologies, among them *Best American Science Writing* (2005).

Ackerman is currently a senior fellow at the Tisch College of Citizenship and Public Service at Tufts University. She has lectured at Harvard University, MIT, the University of Virginia Medical Center, the American Association of University Women, and for numerous other groups and organizations. Born in 1959, she was educated at Yale University, where she graduated cum laude in 1980 with a BA in English. Ackerman is married to novelist Karl Ackerman and has two daughters.

ABOUT TWELVE

TWELVE

TWELVE was established in August 2005 with the objective of publishing no more than one book per month. We strive to publish the singular book, by authors who have a unique perspective and compelling authority. Works that explain our culture; that illuminate, inspire, provoke, and entertain. We seek to establish communities of conversation surrounding our books. Talented authors deserve attention not only from publishers, but from readers as well. To sell the book is only the beginning of our mission. To build avid audiences of readers who are enriched by these works—that is our ultimate purpose.

For more information about forthcoming TWELVE books, please go to www.twelvebooks.com.